THE ADVANCED LOW FODMAP COOKBOOK

Innovative Recipes for IBS Relief and Digestive Health

Daniel N. Tenney

Table of Content

Contents

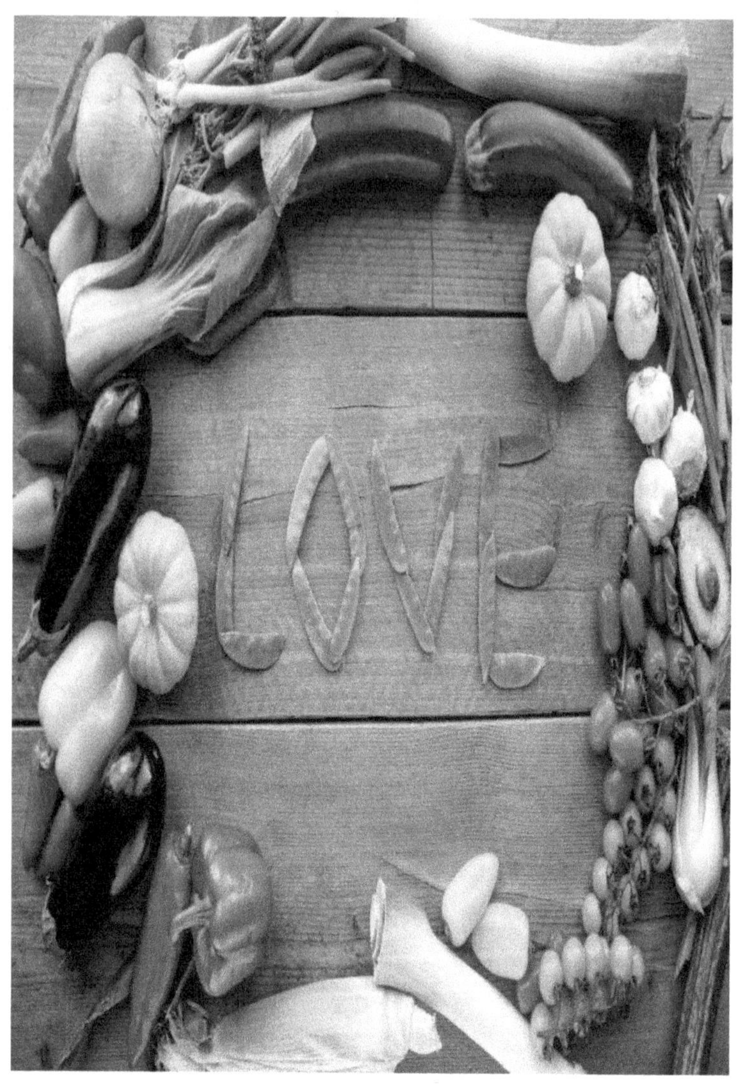

LOVE

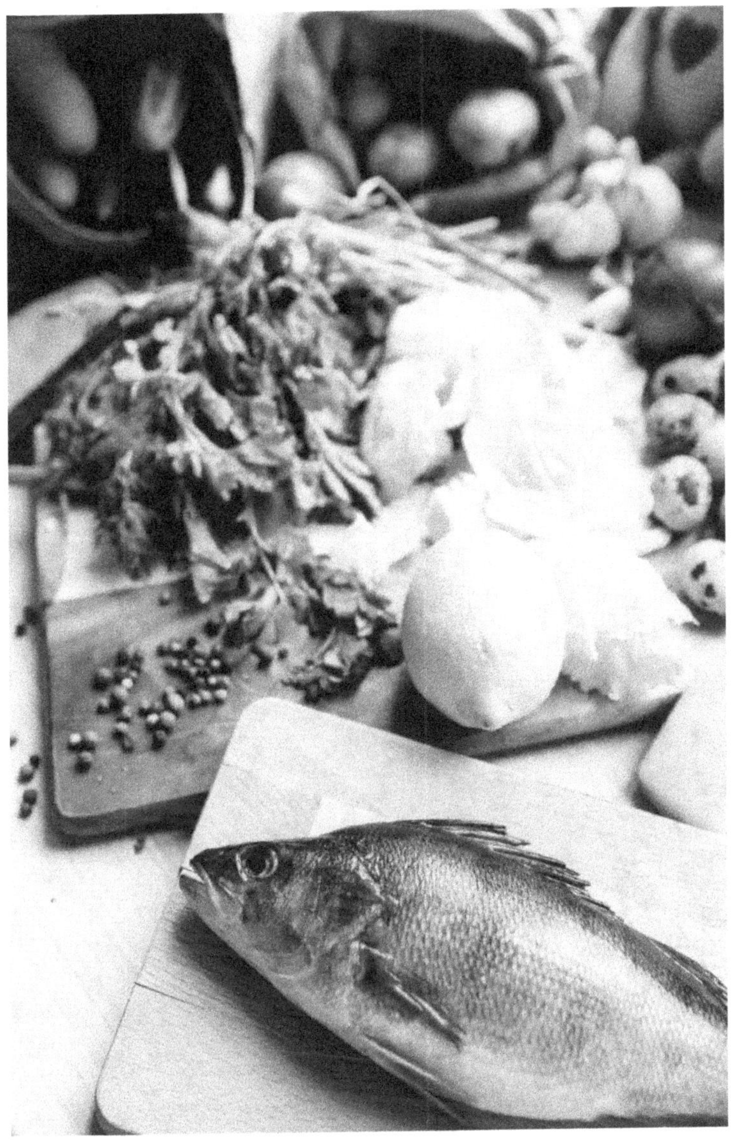

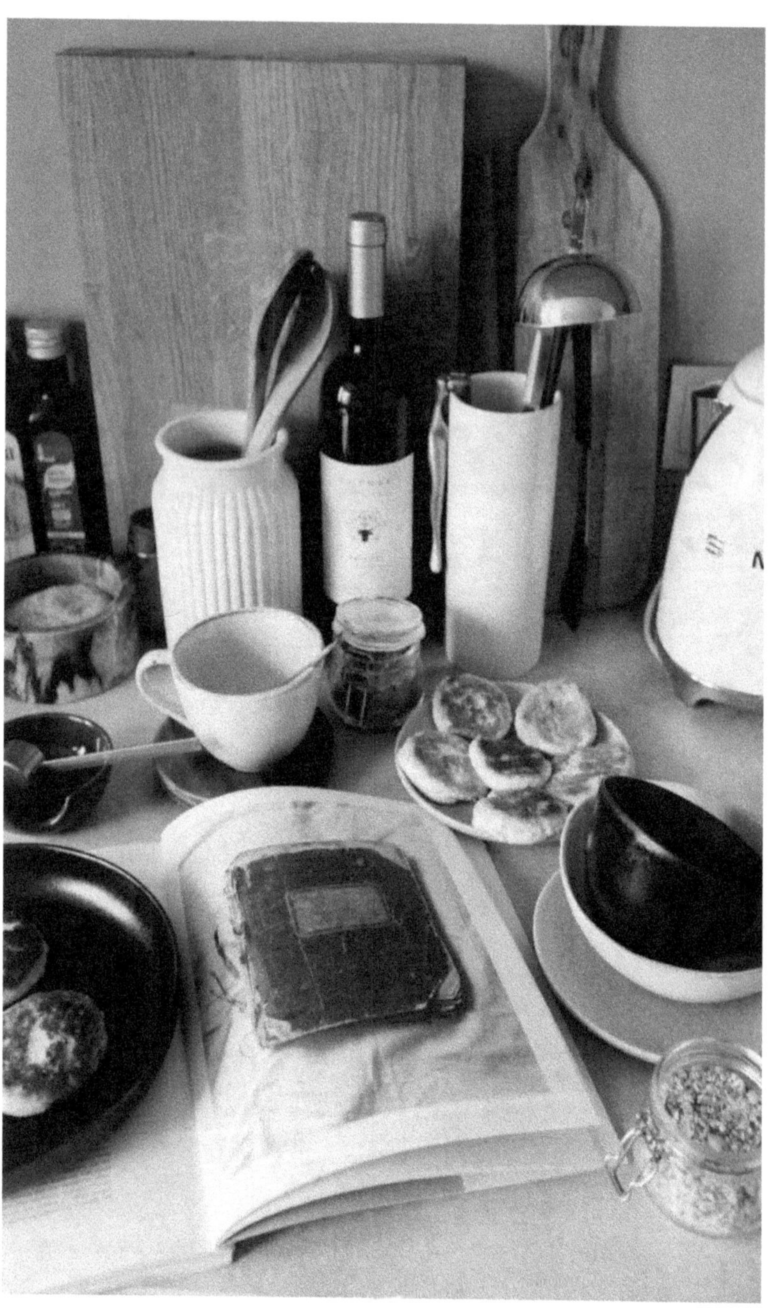

Introduction

Living with Irritable Bowel Syndrome (IBS) can be a daily struggle. The pain and the discomfort can be overwhelming, and there is constant concern about food choices. For many individuals, including myself, finding relief and being able to enjoy meals may seem like a distant dream. That is where the Low FODMAP diet comes in. IBS is a common digestive complaint that affects millions of people worldwide. Symptoms like abdominal pain, bloating, gas, diarrhea, and constipation can significantly impact one's quality of life. The Low FODMAP diet, developed by experimenters at Monash University, offers a result by reducing specific types of carbohydrates that are difficult to digest. By following this diet numerous people with IBS can manage their symptoms and enjoy a better quality of life. My trip into writing this cookbook began with a particular struggle. Many years ago, I was diagnosed with IBS. The symptoms were enervating, and I was constantly anxious about what to eat. Social gatherings and indeed simple family reflections came with stressful events. I tried colorful diets and specifics, but nothing worked. Also, I discovered the Low FODMAP diet. It was not an instant cure, but slowly, I noticed advancements. I started to feel more and recaptured my love for cuisine and experimenting in the kitchen. As I explored new fashions and acclimated my favorite dishes to fit the Low FODMAP guidelines, I realized that there was a lack of innovative and succulent options for people like me. That is when I decided to produce" The Advanced Low FODMAP Cookbook; Innovative Recipes for IBS Relief and Digestive Health." This book is a collection of incredible recipes that aren't only Low FODMAP but also delicious and instigative. I wanted to show that managing IBS does not mean giving up on the joy of eating. In this cookbook, you will find a variety of recipes, from breakfast delights and hearty meals to amazing sauces and international flavors. Each form is designed to be easy to follow and packed with flavor, making it easier to stick to the Low FODMAP diet and enjoy your refections without solicitude. This cookbook encourages you to reclaim authority over your digestive and rediscover the pleasure of eating. The journey may not always be easy, but with the right tools and a bit of creativity, you can manage your IBS and live a fuller, happier life. So, let's embark on this trip together. Savor the content of this cookbook, experiment in your kitchen, and most importantly, enjoy the process. I encourage you to read on and take the first step towards better digestive health and culinary adventures.

Chapter One: Unraveling the Mysteries of the Low FODMAP Diet.

The Origins of FODMAPs

Researchers at Monash University in Australia first proposed the notion of FODMAPs (fermentable oligosaccharides, disaccharides, monosaccharides, and polyols) in the early 2000s. Led by Professor Peter Gibson, the team investigated the link between nutrition and irritable bowel syndrome (IBS) and discovered that particular carbs appeared to cause symptoms in some people.

The researchers hypothesized that these carbohydrates were poorly absorbed in the small intestine and then fermented by bacteria in the large intestine, resulting in gas and other symptoms associated with IBS. They identified four types of carbohydrates that appeared to be especially problematic: oligosaccharides, disaccharides, monosaccharides, and polyols. To test this notion, the researchers conducted a series of tests in which subjects were fed meals with either high or low FODMAPs. They discovered that people who ate low-FODMAP meals had fewer IBS symptoms than those who ate high-FODMAP meals. Since then, the Low FODMAP diet has been a common therapeutic option for people with IBS and other functional gastrointestinal disorders. This diet consists of restricting meals rich in FODMAPs and then gradually reintroducing them to determine which specific carbohydrates are problematic for each individual.

Numerous scientists have supported the hypothesis of FODMAPs. For example, a systematic review and meta-analysis published in the Journal of Gastroenterology and Hepatology found that a low-FODMAP diet effectively reduced IBS symptoms compared to a control diet. Another study published in the American Journal of Gastroenterology found that a low-FODMAP diet improved quality of life and reduced symptoms in people with functional gastrointestinal disorders.

In summary, researchers at Monash University in Australia created the notion of FODMAPs while examining the link between diet and IBS. They identified four types of carbohydrates that appeared to be more harmful to some people and created the Low FODMAP diet as a therapy option. Numerous studies have now backed the diet, and it has emerged as a common therapy choice for people suffering from functional gastrointestinal diseases.

Is low FODMAP scientifically proven?

Numerous studies have shown that the Low FODMAP diet is effective for managing IBS symptoms. A comprehensive review and meta-analysis published in the Journal of Gastroenterology and Hepatology found that a low FODMAP diet was effective in lowering IBS symptoms when compared to a control diet. Another comprehensive review and meta-analysis published in the American Journal of

Gastroenterology discovered that a Low FODMAP diet improved IBS symptoms such as stomach discomfort, bloating, and overall quality of life when compared to a control diet.

The Low FODMAP diet has also been shown to be useful in managing symptoms of various functional gastrointestinal disorders, including functional dyspepsia and functional constipation. According to a controlled trial published in the Journal of Human Nutrition and Dietetics, a low-FODMAP diet relieved functional dyspepsia symptoms more than a control diet did. Another randomized controlled experiment published in the Journal of Gastroenterology and Hepatology discovered that a low-FODMAP diet relieved symptoms of functional constipation when compared to a standard diet.

Several respected organizations, including the American College of Gastroenterology and the British Dietetic Association, have acknowledged the Low FODMAP diet's efficacy. The American College of Gastroenterology advises a low-FODMAP diet as a first-line treatment for IBS, whereas the British

Dietetic Association endorses the use of the Low FODMAP diet to manage IBS symptoms.

It is critical to underline that the Low FODMAP diet is not a one-size-fits-all approach and must be adapted to each person's specific needs and tolerance levels. It is also recommended to work with a qualified dietitian who is familiar with the Low FODMAP diet to ensure optimal nutrition and application.

The connection between low FODMAP and digestive health.

The link between low FODMAP and digestive health stems from the fact that FODMAPs are known to cause symptoms in people with functional gastrointestinal disorders. Reducing your consumption of these carbohydrates reduces the amount of fermentation in your stomach, leading to fewer symptoms. It is crucial to note that the Low FODMAP diet is not all-encompassing and should be tailored to each individual's specific needs and tolerance levels. While the Low FODMAP diet is successful at improving digestive issues, it is not without drawbacks. If not carefully planned and performed, the diet can be restrictive and result in nutrient deficits. However, it is crucial to highlight that, while the diet might be beneficial, it also presents obstacles. The restriction of high-FODMAP foods can reduce prebiotics, which is necessary for the nutrition of good bacteria in the digestive tract. As a result, the concentration of Bifidobacterium, which is essential for gut health, may decrease. As a result, it is recommended that you follow the Low FODMAP diet. As new evidence emerges, the Low FODMAP diet remains an effective strategy for improving digestive health and general quality of life. It allows many people to re-engage in social activities, work more productively, and eat a wider variety of foods with confidence.

Separating Myths from Reality

Low FODMAP diets have grown in popularity in recent years, but they have also resulted in a lot of misinformation and myths. In this part, we'll separate fact from fiction and tell you everything you need to know about this game-changing method of maintaining digestive health. Prepare to have your preconceived beliefs questioned and your knowledge increased as we dispel some of the most popular fallacies about the Low FODMAP diet and offer you the information you need to succeed on this journey.

Myths	Reality
The Low FODMAP diet is a gluten-free diet.	While many gluten-containing foods are high in FODMAPs the Low FODMAP diet is not the same as a gluten-free diet. Gluten is a protein found in wheat barley, and rye, while FODMAPs are carbohydrates found in a variety of foods.
The Low FODMAP diet is a dairy-free diet.	Low FODMAP is not a dairy-free product but a diet-limiting lactose-containing food. unless you have a dairy

	allergy, you don't have to completely avoid dairy altogether.
The Low FODMAP diet is a lifetime diet.	The Low FODMAP diet is not meant to be followed long-term, it's a temporary, learning diet. It is a three-phase approach involving restriction, reintroduction, and personalization to identify individual tolerance levels and create a balanced diet.
The Low FODMAP is a low-carb diet	The Low FODMAP diet is not a low-carb diet. Many high-carbohydrate foods such as fruits and vegetables are allowed on the diet in appropriate proportions.
The Low FODMAP diet is too restrictive.	While the Low FODMAP diet involves restricting certain foods, it is not overly restrictive, many

	nutritious and delicious foods are allowed on the diet, and the reintroduction phase allows for gradually adding foods back into the diet.

It is essential to distinguish between myths and reality regarding the Low FODMAP diet. Having a clear understanding of the facts related to this dietary approach can enable individuals to make well-informed decisions about their health and overall well-being. By dispelling common misconceptions and providing accurate information, we aim to empower individuals to make informed choices about their dietary patterns and enhance their quality of life.

Chapter 2: Breakfast Delight

Smoothies and Shakes

As we discussed in the last chapter, the Low FODMAP diet is an effective tool for addressing digestive health disorders, such as IBS. However, adopting a restricted diet can make meal preparation difficult, particularly during breakfast. Fortunately, several delicious and nutrient filled Low FODMAP breakfast options can assist with IBS symptoms and digestive health. In this chapter, we will introduce breakfast options that are not only low in FODMAPs, but also simple to prepare and full of taste. Whether you're new to the Low FODMAP diet or looking for new breakfast ideas, these recipes are sure to satisfy your taste buds while also benefiting your digestion. We'll look at some delicious and nutritious smoothie and shake options for folks with IBS and other digestive difficulties.

Smoothies and Shakes

Tropical Green Smoothie

Ingredients:

- 1 cup lactose-free yogurt
- 1/2 cup spinach
- 1/2 banana (unripe)
- 1/2 cup pineapple chunks
- 1 tablespoon chia seeds
- 1 cup almond milk

Instructions

1. Combine all ingredients in a blender.
2. Blend until smooth.
3. Pour into a glass and enjoy immediately.

Tip: Unripe bananas are lower in FODMAPs compared to ripe ones, making them a better choice for IBS sufferers.

2. Spicy Sunrise

Ingredients

- 1 cup lactose-free milk
- ½ cup of chopped strawberries
- ¼ cup of lactose-free cottage cheese
- A handful of baby spinach

- A pinch of salt
- Squeeze of lime juice
- Pinch of ground ginger

Instructions

1. Combine all ingredients in a blender. Blend until smooth and vibrant.
2. Enjoy the invigorating blend of sweet, tangy, and spicy flavors!

3. Berry Banana Shake

Ingredients

- 1/2 cup strawberries
- 1/2 cup blueberries
- 1/2 unripe banana
- 1 cup lactose-free milk
- 1 tablespoon flaxseed meal

Instructions

1. Add all ingredients to a blender.
2. Blend until smooth.
3. Serve cold.

Tip: Berries are generally Low FODMAP friendly and add a burst of flavor and antioxidants to your shake.

❖ Quick and Easy Breakfasts

Overnight Oats

Ingredients

- 1/2 cup gluten-free oats
- 1/2 cup lactose-free yogurt
- 1/2 cup almond milk
- 1 tablespoon maple syrup
- 1/4 cup blueberries

Instructions

1. Combine oats, yogurt, and almond milk in a jar.
2. Stir in the maple syrup and blueberries.
3. Refrigerate overnight.
4. In the morning, stir it and enjoy it cold.

Tip: Preparing breakfast, the night before saves time and ensures you have a healthy meal ready to go.

2. Scrambled Eggs with Spinach

Ingredients

- 2 eggs
- 1/2 cup spinach
- 1 tablespoon lactose-free milk
- Salt and pepper to taste
- 1 tablespoon olive oil

Instructions

1. Beat the eggs with lactose-free milk, salt, and pepper.
2. Heat olive oil in a non-stick pan over medium heat.
3. Add spinach and cook until wilted.
4. Pour in the eggs and cook, stirring gently until set.
5. Serve immediately.

Tip: Spinach is a great Low FODMAP vegetable that adds nutrients and color to your breakfast.

3. Low-FODMAP Breakfast Burrito Bowl:

Prep Time: 10 minutes

Ingredients

- eggs (scrambled)

- Splash of lactose-free milk
- ½ cup cooked black beans (rinsed and drained)
- Chopped avocado
- Salsa
- Lactose-free sour cream (optional)
- Chopped cilantro (optional)

Instructions:

1. Scramble two eggs with a splash of lactose-free milk and your favorite spices. Set aside.
2. In a bowl, layer cooked black beans, chopped avocado, and salsa.
3. Top with your scrambled eggs and a dollop of lactose-free sour cream (optional).
4. Finish with a sprinkle of chopped cilantro for a fresh touch.

❖ Hearty Morning Meals

Sweet Potato Hash

Ingredients

- 1 medium sweet potato, diced

- 1/2 bell pepper, diced
- 1/2 zucchini, diced
- 1 tablespoon olive oil
- 1 teaspoon paprika
- Salt and pepper to taste

Instructions

- Heat olive oil in a large pan over medium-high heat.
- Add sweet potato and cook until it starts to soften.
- Add bell pepper, zucchini, paprika, salt, and pepper.
- Cook until all vegetables are tender and slightly crispy.
- Serve hot.

Tip: Sweet potatoes are a great source of fiber and vitamins and are Low FODMAP when eaten in moderation.

Low-FODMAP Frittata

Ingredients

- ½ cup chopped bell peppers (red, yellow, or

orange)

- Handful of chopped spinach
- Drizzle of olive oil
- 6 eggs
- Splash of lactose-free milk
- Grated Parmesan cheese (optional)
- Salt and pepper to taste
- Chopped fresh herbs (optional: chives, parsley, basil)

Instructions

1. Preheat your oven to 375°F (190°C). Grease a non-stick oven-safe pan or pie dish.
2. Heat olive oil in a pan over medium heat. Add chopped bell peppers and spinach. Sauté for 5 minutes, or until softened. Season with a pinch of salt and pepper.
3. In a large bowl, whisk together eggs, a splash of lactose-free milk, and grated Parmesan cheese (if using). Season generously with salt and pepper.
4. Pour the egg mixture into the preheated pan over the sauteed vegetables. Tilt the pan to allow the uncooked egg to fill the gaps.

5. Sprinkle the top with your favorite chopped fresh herbs (optional).

6. Bake in the preheated oven for 20-25 minutes, or until the eggs are set and the center is no longer runny. A toothpick inserted in the center should come out clean.

7. Let the frittata cool slightly before slicing and serving. Enjoy warm with a side of lactose-free yogurt and berries.

3. Low-FODMAP Breakfast Tacos

Prep Time: 10 minutes (cook) + assembly time

Ingredients

- ½ cup ground turkey (or crumbled tempeh for a vegetarian option)
- Taco seasoning (low-FODMAP brand)
- 2 low-FODMAP corn tortillas (check serving size)
- Chopped tomatoes
- Shredded lettuce
- Lactose-free sour cream (optional)
- Chopped avocado (optional)
- Salsa

- Chopped cilantro (optional)

Instructions

1. In a pan over medium heat, cook a ground turkey (or tempeh) according to package instructions, breaking it up with a spatula as it cooks. Season with taco seasoning.
2. Warm your low-FODMAP corn tortillas according to package instructions (usually by wrapping them in a damp paper towel and microwaving for 30 seconds).
3. Assemble your breakfast tacos! Fill each tortilla with seasoned ground turkey/tempeh, chopped tomatoes, shredded lettuce, and your favorite toppings like lactose-free sour cream, chopped avocado, salsa, and chopped cilantro.

Quinoa Breakfast Bowl

Ingredients

- 1/2 cup cooked quinoa
- 1/2 avocado, sliced
- 1 egg
- 1/4 cup cherry tomatoes, halved
- 1 tablespoon olive oil
- Salt and pepper to taste

Instructions

1. Cook quinoa according to package instructions.
2. Heat olive oil in a pan over medium heat and fry the egg to your liking.
3. Assemble the bowl: quinoa at the base, topped with avocado, cherry tomatoes, and the fried egg.
4. Season with salt and pepper.

Tip: Quinoa is a great gluten-free grain that provides protein and is easy on the digestive system.

Feel free to customize your fillings and toppings based on your preferences and what your gut tolerates! Let's move on to the next chapter and discover more delightful Low FODMAP recipes!

Chapter 3: Snacks and Appetizers

Snacks and appetizers are essential parts of any diet, providing quick energy boosts and satisfying small cravings throughout the day. For those following a Low FODMAP diet, it's important to have a variety of delicious and easy-to-make options. Here are some tasty, Low FODMAP-friendly recipes for light bites, party pleasers, and healthy munchies.

Light Bites for Any Time

Cucumber and Dill Hummus Bites

Ingredients

- 1 cucumber, sliced into rounds
- 1 cup canned chickpeas, rinsed and drained
- 2 tablespoons tahini
- 1 tablespoon lemon juice
- 1 tablespoon olive oil
- 1 teaspoon dried dill
- Salt and pepper to taste

Directions

1. In a food processor, blend the chickpeas, tahini, lemon juice, olive oil, and dill until smooth.
2. Season with salt and pepper.
3. Place a dollop of hummus on each cucumber slice.
4. Garnish with a sprinkle of dill and serve.

Tip: Keep the cucumber slices in the fridge until you're ready to serve for a refreshing bite.

2. Caprese Skewers with a Twist

Ingredients

- ½ cup cherry tomatoes (halved or quartered)
- ½ cup lactose-free mozzarella pearls
- ½ cup fresh basil leaves
- ¼ cup extra virgin olive oil
- 1 tablespoon balsamic vinegar
- Pinch of dried oregano
- Salt and pepper to taste
- Bamboo skewers

Instructions

1. In a small bowl, whisk together olive oil, balsamic vinegar, oregano, salt, and pepper.

2. Thread cherry tomatoes, mozzarella pearls, and basil leaves alternately onto bamboo skewers.

3. Drizzle the skewers with the prepared vinaigrette.

4. Serve immediately or refrigerate for up to 30 minutes for a chilled and refreshing bite.

Tip: Want to add a protein boost? Thread some grilled chicken or shrimp onto the skewers for a heartier option.

3. Edamame with a Zing

Ingredients

- 2 cups shelled edamame (fresh or frozen)
- 1 tablespoon olive oil
- ½ teaspoon ground ginger
- ½ teaspoon garlic powder (check for low-FODMAP brand)
- Pinch of red pepper flakes (optional)

- Sea salt to taste

Instructions

1. If using frozen edamame, cook according to package instructions. For fresh edamame, blanch in boiling water for 3-4 minutes, then drain and rinse with cold water.
2. Heat olive oil in a pan over medium heat. Add ginger and garlic powder, and cook for 30 seconds, releasing the aromatics.
3. Add edamame and toss to coat. Cook for another minute or two, until heated through.
4. Sprinkle with red pepper flakes (optional) and sea salt to taste.

Tip: Feeling fancy? Drizzle your edamame with a touch of low-FODMAP soy sauce or a sprinkle of furikake for extra umami flavor.

4. Mini Rice Paper Spring Rolls with Peanut Dipping Sauce

Ingredients

- 6-8 rice paper wrappers
- 1 cup lettuce leaves, shredded

- ½ cup julienned cucumber
- ½ cup julienned bell pepper (red, yellow, or orange)
- ½ cup shredded carrots
- Cooked shrimp or chicken (optional, shredded)
- Fresh herbs like mint and cilantro (optional)

For the Peanut Dipping Sauce:

- ¼ cup creamy peanut butter (check for low-FODMAP brand)
- 2 tablespoons low-FODMAP soy sauce
- 1 tablespoon rice vinegar
- 1 tablespoon honey or maple syrup
- 1 tablespoon lime juice
- 1 tablespoon water
- Pinch of red pepper flakes (optional)

Instructions

1. Prepare the dipping sauce by whisking together all ingredients in a small bowl. Set aside.
2. Fill a large shallow dish with warm water. Dip one rice paper wrapper into the water for a few

seconds, just until softened. Lay it flat on a plate.

3. Arrange lettuce, cucumber, bell pepper, carrots, and any protein you're using in the center of the wrapper. Top with fresh herbs (optional).

4. Fold the bottom of the wrapper over the filling, then fold in the sides. Tightly roll up the wrapper to create a spring roll. Repeat with remaining wrappers and fillings.

5. Serve immediately with the peanut dipping sauce.

Tip: Get creative with your fillings! Try adding other low-FODMAP options like shredded cabbage, chopped avocado, or crumbled cooked tofu

Party Pleasers

Mini Caprese Skewers

Ingredients

- 20 cherry tomatoes
- 20 small fresh mozzarella balls

- 10 fresh basil leaves, halved
- 2 tablespoons balsamic glaze
- Salt and pepper to taste
- Toothpicks or small skewers

Instructions

1. On each toothpick or skewer, thread a cherry tomato, a mozzarella ball, and a half basil leaf.
2. Arrange the skewers on a platter.
3. Drizzle with balsamic glaze and sprinkle with salt and pepper before serving.

Tip: These skewers can be assembled a few hours in advance and stored in the fridge until party time.

2. Roasted Vegetable Platter with Whipped Feta Dip

Ingredients

- 1 head of broccoli, cut into florets
- 1 red bell pepper, sliced
- 1 yellow bell pepper, sliced
- 1 red onion, cut into wedges
- 1 zucchini, sliced
- 2 tablespoons olive oil
- Salt and pepper to taste

For the Whipped Feta Dip:

- 8 ounces block of feta cheese, crumbled
- ½ cup lactose-free Greek yogurt
- ¼ cup extra virgin olive oil
- 1 tablespoon lemon juice
- 1 garlic clove, minced
- Pinch of dried oregano
- Pinch of red pepper flakes (optional)
- Fresh herbs like mint or parsley, chopped (for garnish)

Instructions:

1. Preheat oven to 400°F (200°C). Line a baking sheet with parchment paper.
2. Toss broccoli florets, bell pepper slices, red onion wedges, and zucchini slices with olive oil, salt, and pepper. Spread vegetables evenly on the prepared baking sheet.
3. Roast for 20-25 minutes, or until vegetables are tender-crisp and slightly browned.
4. While the vegetables roast, prepare the dip. In a food processor, combine crumbled feta cheese, lactose-free Greek yogurt, olive oil,

lemon juice, garlic, oregano, and red pepper flakes (if using). Blend until smooth and creamy.

5. Transfer the dip to a serving bowl and garnish with chopped fresh herbs.

6. Arrange roasted vegetables around the dip on a platter. Serve warm or at room temperature.

Tip: Want to add a protein element? Drizzle the roasted vegetables with balsamic glaze or serve the platter with grilled chicken or shrimp skewers.

3. Mini Gluten-Free Frittata Cups

Ingredients

- 12 large eggs
- ½ cup chopped spinach
- ½ cup chopped mushrooms
- ½ cup chopped bell peppers (any color)
- ¼ cup chopped cherry tomatoes
- ¼ cup crumbled feta cheese (optional)
- Salt and pepper to taste
- 1 tablespoon olive oil
- 12 non-stick muffin cups

Instructions

1. Preheat oven to 375°F (190°C). Grease non-stick muffin cups with olive oil.
2. In a large bowl, whisk together eggs with salt and pepper.
3. Stir in chopped spinach, mushrooms, bell peppers, cherry tomatoes, and feta cheese (if using).
4. Divide the egg mixture evenly among the prepared muffin cups.
5. Bake for 15-20 minutes, or until the egg is set and the centers are no longer runny. A toothpick inserted in the center should come out clean.
6. Let the frittatas cool slightly before serving.

Tip: Get creative with your fillings! Try adding cooked sausage or crumbled cooked chicken for a heartier option. You can also use different low-FODMAP vegetables like chopped zucchini or asparagus.

4. Grilled Steak with Chimichurri Sauce

Ingredients

- 2-3 steaks (your choice of cut, ensure appropriate portion size)
- Olive oil
- Salt and pepper to taste

For the Chimichurri Sauce:

- 1 cup packed fresh parsley leaves, chopped
- ¼ cup chopped fresh oregano leaves
- 2 tablespoons olive oil
- 2 tablespoons red wine vinegar
- 1 garlic clove, minced
- 1 shallot, minced
- Pinch of red pepper flakes (optional)
- Salt and pepper to taste

Instructions

1. Prepare the chimichurri sauce by combining all ingredients in a bowl. Set aside.
2. Preheat your grill to medium-high heat. Season steaks generously with salt and pepper.
3. Grill steaks to your desired doneness (rare, medium-rare, etc.).
4. Let the steaks rest for a few minutes before slicing.

5. Serve grilled steaks with chimichurri sauce on the side.

Tip: Want to add some grilled vegetables? Toss zucchini slices, bell pepper strips, and red onion wedges with olive oil and salt before grilling alongside the steaks.

Healthy Munchies

Roasted Chickpeas

Ingredients

- 1 can chickpeas, rinsed and drained
- 1 tablespoon olive oil
- 1 teaspoon smoked paprika
- 1/2 teaspoon garlic-infused oil
- Salt to taste

Directions

1. Preheat your oven to 400°F (200°C).
2. Pat the chickpeas dry with a paper towel.
3. In a bowl, toss the chickpeas with olive oil, smoked paprika, garlic-infused oil, and salt.
4. Spread the chickpeas on a baking sheet in a

single layer.

5. Roast for 20-30 minutes, shaking the pan halfway through, until crispy.

6. Let cool before serving.

Tip: Store roasted chickpeas in an airtight container for up to a week for a crunchy snack on the go.

2. Carrot and Zucchini Chips

Ingredients

- 2 large carrots
- 2 large zucchinis
- 1 tablespoon olive oil
- Salt and pepper to taste

Directions

1. Preheat your oven to 350°F (175°C).

2. Slice the carrots and zucchinis thinly using a mandolin or a sharp knife.

3. Toss the vegetable slices with olive oil, salt, and pepper.

4. Arrange the slices in a single layer on a baking

sheet lined with parchment paper.

5. Bake for 15-20 minutes, turning once, until crisp.

6. Allow to cool before serving.

Tip: Keep an eye on the chips as they bake to prevent burning, and store any leftovers in an airtight container to maintain their crunch.

3. Spiced Trail Mix with a Twist

Ingredients

- ½ cup raw almonds (or a mix of low-FODMAP nuts like cashews and macadamia nuts)
- ¼ cup dried cranberries
- ¼ cup puffed quinoa
- 2 tablespoons dark chocolate chips (check for low-FODMAP brands)
- ½ teaspoon ground cinnamon
- ¼ teaspoon ground ginger
- Pinch of ground cardamom

Instructions

1. In a large bowl, combine almonds, dried cranberries, puffed quinoa, and dark chocolate chips.
2. In a small bowl, mix the cinnamon, ginger, and cardamom. Sprinkle the spice mixture over the trail mix and toss to coat.
3. Store in an airtight container for up to a week.

Tip: Want a sweeter option? Drizzle the trail mix with a touch of melted maple syrup or honey before adding the spices.

4. Roasted Chickpea Snack with Herbs

Ingredients

- 1 can chickpeas, drained and rinsed
- 1 tablespoon olive oil
- ½ teaspoon dried rosemary
- ½ teaspoon dried thyme
- Pinch of smoked paprika
- Salt and pepper to taste

Instructions

1. Preheat the oven to 400°F (200°C). Line a baking sheet with parchment paper.
2. Pat the chickpeas dry with a clean kitchen towel.
3. In a bowl, toss chickpeas with olive oil, rosemary, thyme, paprika, salt, and pepper.
4. Spread the chickpeas evenly on the prepared baking sheet.
5. Roast for 20-25 minutes, or until the chickpeas are golden brown and crispy.
6. Let the chickpeas cool slightly before enjoying them.

Tip: Play with different flavor combinations! Try adding a sprinkle of chili powder for a kick, or a dash of curry powder for an Indian-inspired twist.

5. FODMAP-Friendly Fruit & Yogurt Parfait

Ingredients

- ½ cup lactose-free yogurt (plain or vanilla)
- ½ cup sliced strawberries
- ¼ cup blueberries
- ¼ cup granola (check for low-FODMAP brands)

- Drizzle of honey or maple syrup (optional)
- Fresh mint leaves (for garnish)

Instructions

1. In a small glass or jar, layer yogurt, sliced strawberries, blueberries, and granola. Repeat layers if desired.
2. Drizzle with a touch of honey or maple syrup (optional) for extra sweetness.
3. Garnish with a fresh mint leaf.

Tip: Feeling fancy? Toast some sliced almonds or chopped walnuts to add a nutty crunch to your parfait.

Conclusion

These snacks and appetizers are perfect for any occasion, whether you need a quick bite, a party treat, or a healthy munch. They're easy to make, delicious, and Low FODMAP-friendly, ensuring you can enjoy them without worrying about your IBS symptoms. Try these recipes out, and feel free to get creative with your variations!

Chapter 4: Soups and Salads

I know sometimes you just crave a warm, comforting bowl of soup or a vibrant salad bursting with fresh flavors. This chapter will equip you with a diverse range of options to suit any palate or occasion while adhering to low FODMAP principles. Each recipe promises a delightful culinary experience that respects your digestive health.

Comforting Soups

Carrot Ginger Soup

Ingredients

- 1 tablespoon olive oil
- 1 pound carrots, peeled and chopped
- 1-inch fresh ginger, peeled and grated
- 4 cups low FODMAP chicken or vegetable broth
- Salt and pepper to taste
- Fresh parsley for garnish

Instructions

1. Heat the olive oil in a large pot over medium heat.

2. Add the chopped carrots and grated ginger. Sauté for about 5 minutes until the carrots start to soften.

3. Pour in the low FODMAP broth and bring to a boil.

4. Reduce the heat and let it simmer for 20 minutes, or until the carrots are tender.

5. Use an immersion blender to puree the soup until smooth. If you don't have an immersion blender, let the soup cool slightly and blend in batches in a regular blender.

6. Season with salt and pepper to taste.

7. Garnish with fresh parsley and serve warm.

Practical Tip: For a creamier texture, you can add a splash of lactose-free cream or coconut milk before blending.

2. Creamy Butternut Squash Soup with Sage

Ingredients

- 1 medium butternut squash, peeled and diced

- 1 tablespoon olive oil
- 1 yellow onion, chopped
- 2 cloves garlic, minced
- 4 cups lactose-free chicken broth
- 1 cup unsweetened lactose-free coconut milk
- ½ cup chopped fresh sage leaves
- Salt and pepper to taste
- Optional garnish: toasted pumpkin seeds and fresh sage leaves

Instructions

1. Heat olive oil in a large pot over medium heat. Add chopped onion and cook until softened about 5 minutes.
2. Add minced garlic and cook for an additional minute, until fragrant.
3. Stir in diced butternut squash and cook for another 2-3 minutes, allowing the squash to release its natural sweetness.
4. Pour in the lactose-free chicken broth and coconut milk. Bring to a boil, then reduce heat and simmer for 20-25 minutes, or until the butternut squash is tender.
5. Remove the pot from heat and stir in fresh sage

leaves. Let the soup sit for 5 minutes to allow the flavors to meld.

6. Using an immersion blender or in batches in a regular blender, puree the soup until smooth and creamy. Season with salt and pepper to taste.

7. Serve hot, garnished with toasted pumpkin seeds and a sprig of fresh sage (optional).

Tip: Want a thicker soup? Reserve some of the diced butternut squash before blending and add it back after pureeing for a bit of chunky texture.

3. Spicy Thai Coconut Curry Noodle Soup

Ingredients

- 1 tablespoon olive oil
- 1 yellow onion, chopped
- 2 cloves garlic, minced
- 1-inch piece of ginger, grated
- 1 red bell pepper, thinly sliced
- 1 green bell pepper, thinly sliced
- 1 tablespoon red curry paste (check for low-

FODMAP brands)

- 4 cups lactose-free vegetable broth
- 1 can (13.5 oz) coconut milk (unsweetened)
- 1 cup chopped broccoli florets
- ½ cup sliced mushrooms
- 1 cup cooked rice noodles (check for low-FODMAP brands)
- 1 tablespoon soy sauce (check for low-FODMAP brands)
- 1 tablespoon lime juice
- Salt and pepper to taste
- Optional garnishes: chopped fresh cilantro, sliced green onions, sriracha

Instructions

1. Heat olive oil in a large pot over medium heat. Add chopped onion and cook until softened about 5 minutes.
2. Stir in minced garlic, grated ginger, and sliced bell peppers. Cook for an additional 2-3 minutes, until fragrant.
3. Add the red curry paste and cook for another minute, allowing the flavors to bloom.
4. Pour in the lactose-free vegetable broth and

coconut milk. Bring to a boil, then reduce heat and simmer for 10 minutes.

5. Add chopped broccoli florets and sliced mushrooms. Simmer for another 5-7 minutes, or until the vegetables are tender-crisp.

6. Stir in cooked rice noodles, soy sauce, and lime juice. Season with salt and pepper to taste.

7. Serve hot, garnished with chopped fresh cilantro, sliced green onions, and a drizzle of sriracha (optional) for extra heat.

Tip: Want to add some protein? This soup is delicious with shredded cooked chicken or shrimp.

4. Chicken and Quinoa Soup

Ingredients

- 1 tablespoon olive oil
- 1 pound boneless, skinless chicken breasts, cut into small pieces
- 1 cup chopped carrots
- 1 cup chopped zucchini

- 1/2 cup quinoa, rinsed
- 6 cups low FODMAP chicken broth
- 1 teaspoon dried thyme
- Salt and pepper to taste
- Fresh parsley for garnish

Directions

1. Heat the olive oil in a large pot over medium heat.
2. Add the chicken pieces and cook until browned.
3. Add the chopped carrots and zucchini, and sauté for another 5 minutes.
4. Stir in the quinoa and pour in the low-FODMAP chicken broth.
5. Add the dried thyme, and bring the soup to a boil.
6. Reduce the heat and let it simmer for 20 minutes, or until the quinoa is cooked and the vegetables are tender.
7. Season with salt and pepper to taste.
8. Garnish with fresh parsley and serve hot.

Practical Tip: Quinoa is a great low-FODMAP grain

that adds protein and texture to the soup. Make sure to rinse it well to remove any bitter coating.

Fresh and Flavorful Salads

Spinach and Strawberry Salad

Ingredients

- 4 cups baby spinach leaves
- 1 cup sliced strawberries
- 1/4 cup crumbled feta cheese (lactose-free)
- 1/4 cup chopped walnuts
- 2 tablespoons balsamic vinegar
- 2 tablespoons olive oil
- Salt and pepper to taste

Directions

1. In a large bowl, combine the baby spinach, sliced strawberries, crumbled feta cheese, and chopped walnuts.
2. In a small bowl, whisk together the balsamic vinegar and olive oil. Season with salt and pepper.
3. Drizzle the dressing over the salad and toss gently to combine.

4. Serve immediately.

Practical Tip: To keep the salad fresh, add the dressing just before serving. You can also swap walnuts for sunflower seeds if you prefer.

2. Quinoa and Veggie Salad

Ingredients

- 1 cup cooked quinoa
- 1 cup cherry tomatoes, halved
- 1 cup cucumber, diced
- 1/4 cup chopped green onions (green tops only)
- 2 tablespoons fresh lemon juice
- 2 tablespoons olive oil
- Salt and pepper to taste
- Fresh parsley for garnish

Directions

1. In a large bowl, combine the cooked quinoa, cherry tomatoes, cucumber, and green onions.
2. In a small bowl, whisk together the fresh lemon juice and olive oil. Season with salt and pepper.

3. Pour the dressing over the quinoa mixture and toss to combine.

4. Garnish with fresh parsley and serve.

Tip: This salad can be made ahead of time and stored in the refrigerator. It's perfect for meal prep and stays fresh for up to three days.

3. Mediterranean Quinoa Salad with Lemon Vinaigrette

Ingredients

- ¼ cup chopped fresh parsley
- For the Lemon Vinaigrette:
    - ¼ cup extra virgin olive oil
    - 2 tablespoons lemon juice
    - 1 tablespoon rice vinegar (check for low-FODMAP brands)
    - 1 teaspoon dried oregano
    - ½ teaspoon honey
    - Pinch of salt and pepper

Instructions

1. In a large bowl, combine cooked quinoa, chopped cucumber, halved cherry tomatoes, crumbled feta cheese (if using), Kalamata

olives, red onion, and fresh parsley.

2. To make the lemon vinaigrette, whisk together olive oil, lemon juice, rice vinegar, oregano, honey, salt, and pepper in a small bowl.

3. Pour the vinaigrette over the salad ingredients and toss to coat.

4. Serve immediately or refrigerate for up to 30 minutes for chilled flavors.

Tip: Want to add some protein? Toss in some grilled chicken, shrimp, or baked tofu cubes for a heartier salad.

4. Asian Noodle Salad with Peanut Dressing

This vibrant salad is a flavor explosion with a touch of crunch.

Ingredients

- 2 cups rice noodles (check for low-FODMAP brands), cooked according to package instructions
- 1 cup shredded carrots
- ½ cup chopped red bell pepper
- ½ cup sliced sugar snap peas

- ¼ cup chopped fresh cilantro

- ¼ cup chopped roasted peanuts

For the Peanut Dressing:

- ¼ cup creamy peanut butter (check for low-FODMAP brands)

- 2 tablespoons low-FODMAP soy sauce

- 1 tablespoon rice vinegar (check for low-FMAP brands)

- 1 tablespoon lime juice

- 1 tablespoon honey or maple syrup

- 1 tablespoon sriracha (optional)

- 1 clove garlic, minced

- 1-inch ginger, grated

- Water (to thin, as needed)

Instructions

1. Cook rice noodles according to package instructions and drain. Rinse with cold water to stop the cooking process.

2. In a large bowl, combine cooked rice noodles,

shredded carrots, chopped red bell pepper, sliced sugar snap peas, and chopped fresh cilantro.

3. To make the peanut dressing, whisk together peanut butter, soy sauce, rice vinegar, lime juice, honey or maple syrup, sriracha (if using), minced garlic, and grated ginger in a small bowl. Add a tablespoon of water at a time to thin the dressing to the desired consistency.

4. Pour the peanut dressing over the salad ingredients and toss to coat.

5. Garnish with chopped roasted peanuts and serve immediately.

Tip: Want to add some protein? Consider adding grilled chicken or tofu for a more complete meal.

❖ **Dressings & Toppings:**

Lemon Herb Vinaigrette

Ingredients

- ¼ cup extra virgin olive oil
- 2 tablespoons lemon juice
- 1 tablespoon balsamic vinegar
- 1 teaspoon Dijon mustard

- 1 teaspoon dried oregano
- ½ teaspoon dried thyme
- Pinch of salt and pepper

Instructions

1. In a small jar or container with a lid, whisk together olive oil, lemon juice, balsamic vinegar, Dijon mustard, oregano, thyme, salt, and pepper.
2. Shake well to emulsify the dressing.
3. Store in the refrigerator for up to a week. Shake well before using.

Tip: Want to add a garlic kick? Mince a garlic clove and add it to the dressing before shaking.

2. Creamy Avocado Cilantro Dressing

Ingredients

- ½ ripe avocado peeled and pitted
- ¼ cup chopped fresh cilantro
- 2 tablespoons lime juice

- 1 tablespoon olive oil
- 1 tablespoon low-FODMAP yogurt (optional)
- Salt and pepper to taste

Instructions

1. In a blender or food processor, combine avocado, chopped cilantro, lime juice, olive oil, and yogurt (if using).
2. Blend until smooth and creamy. Season with salt and pepper to taste.
3. Serve immediately or store in the refrigerator for up to 2 days.

Tip: Want a thinner consistency? Add a tablespoon of water or lactose-free milk to the dressing before blending.

3. Lemon Herb Dressing

Ingredients:

- 1/4 cup fresh lemon juice
- 1/4 cup olive oil
- 1 teaspoon Dijon mustard
- 1 tablespoon chopped fresh basil
- Salt and pepper to taste

Directions

1. In a small bowl, whisk together the lemon juice, olive oil, and Dijon mustard.
2. Stir in the chopped basil and season with salt and pepper.
3. Drizzle over your favorite salad or use as a marinade for grilled vegetables.

Practical Tip: Fresh herbs add a burst of flavor to any dressing. Feel free to experiment with different herbs like cilantro, parsley, or dill.

With these soups and salads, you have a variety of options to keep your meals exciting and IBS-friendly. Enjoy these recipes, and don't hesitate to experiment by adding your favorite Low FODMAP ingredients. Happy cooking!

Chapter 5: Poultry Perfection

Welcome to the chapter on Poultry Perfection! In this

chapter, we'll explore delicious, Low FODMAP poultry recipes that are easy to make and packed with flavor. Whether you prefer chicken or turkey, you'll find something here to satisfy your taste buds. Let's get started!

Chicken Dishes

Lemon Herb Grilled Chicken

Ingredients

- 4 boneless, skinless chicken breasts
- 2 tablespoons olive oil
- 2 tablespoons fresh lemon juice
- 1 teaspoon dried oregano
- 1 teaspoon dried thyme
- 1 teaspoon salt
- 1/2 teaspoon black pepper

Instructions

1. In a small bowl, mix olive oil, lemon juice, oregano, thyme, salt, and pepper.
2. Place the chicken breasts in a shallow dish and pour the marinade over them. Let it marinate for at least 30 minutes.

3. Preheat the grill to medium-high heat.

4. Grill the chicken for 6-7 minutes on each side or until the internal temperature reaches 165°F (75°C).

5. Serve with your favorite Low FODMAP side dish.

Tip: For even cooking, pound the chicken breasts to an even thickness before marinating.

2. Moroccan Chicken Tagine with Preserved Lemons and Olives

Ingredients

- 1 tablespoon olive oil
- 1 medium onion, chopped
- 2 cloves garlic, minced
- 1 teaspoon ground ginger
- ½ teaspoon ground turmeric
- Pinch of cinnamon
- ½ teaspoon ground coriander
- ¼ teaspoon cayenne pepper (adjust to preference)

- 1 (14.5 oz) can diced tomatoes, undrained
- 1 cup chicken broth (low-FODMAP brand)
- 1 bay leaf
- 2 boneless, skinless chicken breasts
- ½ cup pitted Kalamata olives
- 1 preserved lemon, quartered (rinsed and seeds removed)
- Chopped fresh cilantro, for garnish

Instructions

1. Heat olive oil in a large Dutch oven or heavy-bottomed pot over medium heat. Add chopped onion and cook until softened, about 5 minutes.
2. Stir in minced garlic, ginger, turmeric, cinnamon, coriander, and cayenne pepper. Cook for an additional minute, allowing the aromas to bloom.
3. Pour in the diced tomatoes with their juices, chicken broth, and bay leaf. Bring to a simmer.
4. Season with salt and pepper to taste. Nestle the chicken breasts into the simmering sauce.
5. Add the pitted Kalamata olives and quartered preserved lemon. Reduce heat to low, cover,

and simmer for 20-25 minutes, or until the chicken is cooked through.

6. Remove the chicken from the pot and shred it with two forks. Return the shredded chicken to the sauce.

7. Discard the bay leaf and preserved lemon quarters. Taste and adjust seasonings as needed.

8. Serve the chicken tagine over your favorite low-FODMAP rice or quinoa. Garnish with chopped fresh cilantro.

Tip: Want to add some vegetables? Toss in chopped zucchini, bell peppers, or carrots along with the tomatoes for added color and nutrients.

2. Thai Coconut Curry Chicken with Green Beans

This vibrant curry is packed with flavor and perfect for a satisfying low-FODMAP meal.

Ingredients:

- 1 tablespoon olive oil
- 1 yellow onion, chopped

- 2 cloves garlic, minced
- 1 tablespoon red curry paste (check for low-FODMAP brands)
- 1 (13.5 oz) can coconut milk (unsweetened)
- ½ cup chicken broth (low-FODMAP brand)
- 1 tablespoon soy sauce (check for low-FODMAP brands)
- 1 tablespoon brown sugar
- 1 pound boneless, skinless chicken thighs, cut into bite-sized pieces
- 1 cup trimmed green beans, cut into 1-inch pieces
- Chopped fresh cilantro and lime wedges, for garnish

Instructions

1. Heat olive oil in a large pot or Dutch oven over medium heat. Add chopped onion and cook until softened, about 5 minutes.

2. Stir in minced garlic and red curry paste. Cook for an additional minute, allowing the flavors to release.

3. Pour in the coconut milk, chicken broth, soy sauce, and brown sugar. Bring to a simmer.

4. Add the chicken pieces and simmer for 10-12 minutes, or until the chicken is partially cooked through.

5. Stir in the green beans and simmer for an additional 5-7 minutes, or until the vegetables are tender-crisp and the chicken is cooked through.

6. Serve the Thai coconut curry chicken over your favorite low-FODMAP rice or noodles. Garnish with chopped fresh cilantro and lime wedges.

Tip: Want to add some protein variety? Swap the chicken thighs for shrimp or firm tofu cubes, adjusting cooking times as needed.

3. Baked Garlic Parmesan Chicken

Ingredients:

- 4 boneless, skinless chicken thighs
- 2 tablespoons garlic-infused oil
- 1/2 cup grated Parmesan cheese
- 1 teaspoon paprika
- 1/2 teaspoon salt
- 1/4 teaspoon black pepper

Instructions

1. Preheat your oven to 375°F (190°C).
2. In a bowl, combine Parmesan cheese, paprika, salt, and pepper.
3. Brush the chicken thighs with garlic-infused oil.
4. Coat each thigh with the cheese mixture.
5. Place the chicken on a baking sheet and bake for 25-30 minutes or until golden brown and cooked through.
6. Serve with a side of roasted Low FODMAP vegetables.

Tip: Use a meat thermometer to ensure the chicken reaches an internal temperature of 165°F (75°C).

Turkey Recipes

Turkey Meatballs

Ingredients

- 1 pound ground turkey
- 1/2 cup gluten-free breadcrumbs

- 1/4 cup lactose-free milk
- 1 egg
- 1 tablespoon garlic-infused oil
- 1 teaspoon dried basil
- 1 teaspoon dried oregano
- 1/2 teaspoon salt
- 1/4 teaspoon black pepper

Instructions

1. Preheat your oven to 400°F (200°C).
2. In a large bowl, combine all ingredients and mix well.
3. Form the mixture into 1-inch meatballs and place them on a baking sheet lined with parchment paper.
4. Bake for 20-25 minutes or until the meatballs are cooked through and golden brown.
5. Serve with a Low FODMAP tomato sauce and gluten-free pasta.

Tip: Double the recipe and freeze half of the meatballs for an easy meal later.

2. Herb-Roasted Turkey Breast

Ingredients

- 1 turkey breast (about 2 pounds)
- 2 tablespoons olive oil
- 1 tablespoon fresh rosemary, chopped
- 1 tablespoon fresh thyme, chopped
- 1 teaspoon salt
- 1/2 teaspoon black pepper

Instructions

1. Preheat your oven to 350°F (175°C).
2. In a small bowl, mix olive oil, rosemary, thyme, salt, and pepper.
3. Rub the turkey breast with the herb mixture.
4. Place the turkey breast on a roasting pan and roast for 1-1.5 hours, or until the internal temperature reaches 165°F (75°C).
5. Let the turkey rest for 10 minutes before slicing.
6. Serve with Low FODMAP gravy and your favorite sides.

Tip: Baste the turkey breast with its juices every 20 minutes to keep it moist.

3. Turkey Lettuce Wraps with Peanut Sauce

Instructions

1. Heat a large skillet over medium heat. Add a drizzle of olive oil.
2. Sauté the chopped red bell pepper and green onion for 2-3 minutes, until softened.
3. Add the ground turkey to the pan and cook, breaking it up with a spoon, until browned and cooked through.
4. Stir in the soy sauce, brown sugar, ginger, garlic powder, and red pepper flakes (if using). Cook for an additional minute to allow the flavors to meld.
5. While the turkey mixture cooks, prepare the peanut sauce. In a small bowl, whisk together creamy peanut butter, soy sauce, rice vinegar, honey or maple syrup, lime juice, water, and red pepper flakes (if using).
6. Assemble the lettuce wraps by placing a spoonful of the turkey mixture in each romaine lettuce leaf. Drizzle with peanut sauce and serve immediately.

Tip: Want to add some extra crunch? Top the wraps

with chopped peanuts, shredded carrots, or sliced cucumbers.

4. One-Pan Lemon Herb Turkey and Vegetable Sheet Pan Dinner

Ingredients

- 1 pound boneless, skinless turkey breast or thighs, cut into bite-sized pieces
- 1 tablespoon olive oil
- 1 tablespoon dried oregano
- ½ teaspoon garlic powder
- Salt and pepper to taste
- 1 cup chopped broccoli florets
- 1 cup sliced red bell pepper
- ½ cup chopped zucchini
- Cherry tomatoes (optional)
- 1 lemon, sliced

Instructions

1. Preheat oven to 400°F (200°C).
2. In a large bowl, toss turkey pieces with olive oil, oregano, garlic powder, salt, and pepper.
3. Add chopped broccoli florets, sliced red bell pepper, zucchini, and cherry tomatoes (if

using) to the bowl and toss to coat with the seasonings.

4. Spread the turkey and vegetables evenly on a large baking sheet. Arrange lemon slices over the top.

5. Roast for 25-30 minutes, or until the turkey is cooked through and the vegetables are tender-crisp.

6. Serve immediately.

Tip: Want to add some extra flavor? Drizzle the baking sheet with a splash of chicken broth halfway through cooking to create a pan sauce.

Innovative Poultry Meals

Chicken and Spinach Stuffed Peppers

Ingredients:

- 4 large bell peppers
- 2 cups cooked, shredded chicken

- 1 cup cooked quinoa
- 1 cup fresh spinach, chopped
- 1/2 cup grated Parmesan cheese
- 1 tablespoon garlic-infused oil
- 1 teaspoon dried basil
- 1/2 teaspoon salt
- 1/4 teaspoon black pepper

Instructions

1. Preheat your oven to 375°F (190°C).
2. Cut the tops off the bell peppers and remove the seeds.
3. In a large bowl, combine chicken, quinoa, spinach, Parmesan cheese, garlic-infused oil, basil, salt, and pepper.
4. Stuff the mixture into the bell peppers and place them in a baking dish.
5. Cover with foil and bake for 30 minutes.
6. Remove the foil and bake for an additional 10 minutes, until the peppers are tender and the tops are golden brown.
7. Serve warm.

Tip: Use different colored bell peppers for a visually

appealing dish.

2. Turkey and Zucchini Skillet

Ingredients

- 1 pound ground turkey
- 2 medium zucchinis, diced
- 1 red bell pepper, diced
- 1 tablespoon garlic-infused oil
- 1 teaspoon dried oregano
- 1/2 teaspoon salt
- 1/4 teaspoon black pepper

Instructions

3. For the Ground Turkey Filling

1. Heat garlic-infused oil in a large skillet over medium heat.
2. Add ground turkey and cook until browned, breaking it apart with a spoon.
3. Add diced zucchini, red bell pepper, oregano, salt, and pepper.
4. Cook for another 10 minutes, stirring occasionally, until the vegetables are tender.
5. Serve hot.

Tip: This dish pairs well with a side of cooked quinoa or rice.

4. Deconstructed Shepherd's Pie with Ground Turkey and Sweet Potato

Ingredients

- ½ pound ground turkey
- ½ cup chopped onion
- ½ cup chopped mushrooms
- 1 tablespoon olive oil
- 1 tablespoon tomato paste (check for low-FODMAP brands)
- ½ cup low-FODMAP beef broth
- ½ teaspoon dried thyme
- Salt and pepper to taste

For the Sweet Potato Mash

- 1 medium sweet potato, peeled and diced
- ½ cup water

- 1 tablespoon olive oil

- Salt and pepper to taste

Instructions

1. Preheat oven to 400°F (200°C).

2. In a large skillet, heat olive oil over medium heat. Add chopped onion and cook until softened, about 5 minutes.

3. Stir in chopped mushrooms and cook for an additional 2-3 minutes, until tender.

4. Add the ground turkey to the pan and cook, breaking it up with a spoon, until browned and cooked through.

5. Stir in the tomato paste, beef broth, and thyme. Season with salt and pepper to taste. Simmer for 5 minutes to allow the flavors to meld.

6. While the turkey mixture simmers, prepare the sweet potato mash. In a saucepan, combine diced sweet potato and water. Bring to a boil, then reduce heat and simmer for 15-20 minutes, or until the sweet potato is tender.

7. Drain the water and mash the sweet potato with olive oil, salt, and pepper.

8. To assemble the dish, spoon the ground turkey

mixture into individual serving dishes. Top with the sweet potato mash.

9. Bake for 10-15 minutes, or until the sweet potato mash is slightly golden brown.

10. Serve immediately.

Tip: Want to add some extra texture? Top the dish with a sprinkle of chopped fresh parsley or crispy fried shallots for a delicious finishing touch.

Enjoy these delightful poultry recipes and bring variety to your diet. These dishes are designed to be simple, flavorful, and IBS-friendly, helping you to enjoy meals without worry.

Chapter 6: Fabulous Fish and Seafood

Fish and seafood are excellent sources of lean protein and essential nutrients, making them a great choice for a Low FODMAP diet. In this chapter, we'll explore a variety of delicious and easy-to-make recipes that will make your taste buds dance while keeping your digestive system happy. Whether you prefer quick fish recipes, shellfish delicacies, or special seafood dishes, you'll find something to love here.

Quick Fish Recipes:

Pan-seared cod with Lemon Butter Sauce and Asparagus

Ingredients

- 2 cod fillets (about 6 oz each)
- 1 tablespoon olive oil
- Salt and pepper to taste
- ½ cup chopped asparagus
- 2 tablespoons unsalted butter
- 1 tablespoon lemon juice
- Chopped fresh parsley, for garnish

Instructions

1. Pat the cod fillets dry with paper towels. Season both sides generously with salt and pepper.
2. Heat olive oil in a large skillet over medium-high heat.
3. Sear the cod fillets for 3-4 minutes per side, or until golden brown and cooked through.
4. While the cod cooks, blanch the asparagus in a

pot of boiling water for 2-3 minutes until tender-crisp. Drain and st aside.

5. Once the cod is cooked, remove it from the pan and set aside on a plate.

6. Reduce the heat to low and add the butter to the pan. Let the butter melt and swirl to cook slightly about 30 seconds.

7. Stir in the lemon juice, scraping up any browned bits from the bottom of the pan.

8. Add the blanched asparagus back to the pan and toss to coat with the lemon butter sauce.

9. Plate the cod fillets and top with the asparagus mixture. Drizzle with any remaining pan sauce and garnish with chopped fresh parsley.

Tip: Want to add a touch of heat? Add a pinch of red pepper flakes to the lemon butter sauce.

2. Salmon with Spicy Mango Salsa and Coconut Rice

Ingredients

- 2 salmon fillets (about 6 oz each)
- 1 tablespoon olive oil
- Salt and pepper to taste

For the Spicy Mango Salsa:

- 1 ripe mango, diced
- ½ red bell pepper, diced
- ¼ red onion, diced (rinse with cold water for 10 minutes to reduce harshness)
- 1 jalapeno pepper, seeded and finely chopped (adjust to preference for heat)
- 1 tablespoon chopped fresh cilantro
- 1 tablespoon lime juice
- Salt and pepper to taste

For the Coconut Rice:

- 1 cup jasmine rice
- 1 ½ cups low-FODMAP chicken broth
- 1 (13.5 oz) can unsweetened coconut milk
- ½ teaspoon salt

Instructions

1. Preheat oven to 400°F (200°C).
2. Pat the salmon fillets dry with paper towels. Season both sides generously with salt and pepper.

3. In a baking dish, drizzle the salmon with olive oil. Bake for 15-20 minutes, or until cooked through and flaky.

4. While the salmon cooks, prepare the spicy mango salsa. In a bowl, combine diced mango, red bell pepper, red onion, jalapeno pepper, cilantro, lime juice, and salt and pepper to taste.

5. To make the coconut rice, rinse the jasmine rice in a fine-mesh sieve. In a saucepan, combine the rinsed rice, chicken broth, coconut milk, and salt. Bring to a boil, then reduce heat to low, cover, and simmer for 15-20 minutes, or until the rice is cooked through and fluffy.

6. Serve the baked salmon over a bed of coconut rice and top with the spicy mango salsa.

Tip: Want a vegetarian option? Substitute the salmon with grilled tofu steaks marinated in low-FODMAP teriyaki sauce

3. Herb Baked Salmon

Ingredients:

- 4 salmon fillets
- 2 tablespoons olive oil
- Juice of 1 lemon
- 2 teaspoons dried oregano
- 2 teaspoons dried basil
- Salt and pepper to taste

Instructions

1. Preheat your oven to 375°F (190°C).
2. Place the salmon fillets on a baking sheet lined with parchment paper.
3. In a small bowl, mix olive oil, lemon juice, oregano, basil, salt, and pepper.
4. Brush the mixture over the salmon fillets.
5. Bake for 15-20 minutes, or until the salmon is cooked through and flakes easily with a fork.

Practical Tip: To check if your salmon is done, use a fork to see if it flakes easily. Overcooking can make it dry, so keep an eye on it.

4. Simple Grilled Tilapia

Ingredients

- 4 tilapia fillets

- 2 tablespoons olive oil
- 1 teaspoon paprika
- 1 teaspoon garlic-infused oil (ensure no garlic pieces)
- Salt and pepper to taste

Instructions

1. Preheat your grill to medium-high heat.
2. Brush tilapia fillets with olive oil.
3. Sprinkle paprika, garlic-infused oil, salt, and pepper evenly on both sides.
4. Grill the fillets for 3-4 minutes per side, or until the fish is opaque and flakes easily with a fork.

Practical Tip: Use a fish spatula to flip the fillets to prevent them from breaking apart on the grill.

Shellfish Delicacies

Scallops with Creamy Leek Sauce and Lemon Zest

Ingredients

- 1 pound large sea scallops (dry-packed)
- 1 tablespoon olive oil

- 2 leeks, white and light green parts only, thinly sliced
- 2 garlic cloves, minced
- ½ cup dry white wine (check for low-FODMAP brands)
- ½ cup lactose-free heavy cream
- 1 tablespoon grated lemon zest
- Salt and pepper to taste
- Chopped fresh parsley, for garnish

Instructions

1. Pat the scallops dry with paper towels. Season generously with salt and pepper.
2. Heat olive oil in a large skillet over medium-high heat. Sear the scallops for 2-3 minutes per side, or until golden brown and cooked through (opaque throughout). Remove the scallops from the pan and set aside on a plate.
3. Reduce the heat to medium and add the sliced leeks to the pan. Sauté for 5-7 minutes, or until softened and translucent.
4. Stir in the minced garlic and cook for an additional minute, allowing the aroma to bloom.

5. Pour in the dry white wine and scrape up any browned bits from the bottom of the pan. Simmer for 2-3 minutes, or until the wine has reduced slightly.

6. Add the lactose-free heavy cream and grated lemon zest to the pan. Season with salt and pepper to taste. Bring to a simmer and cook for 2-3 minutes, or until the sauce thickens slightly.

7. Return the cooked scallops back to the pan and spoon the creamy leek sauce over them. Warm them through for an additional minute.

8. Serve the scallops with the creamy leek sauce spooned over the top. Garnish with chopped fresh parsley.

Tip: Want to add a touch of luxury? Serve the scallops and creamy leek sauce over a bed of low-FODMAP risotto or rice pilaf.

2. Garlic-infused Shrimp Scampi

Ingredients

- 1 pound shrimp, peeled and deveined

- 2 tablespoons garlic-infused oil
- 1/4 cup dry white wine
- Juice of 1 lemon
- 2 tablespoons chopped fresh parsley
- Salt and pepper to taste

Instructions

1. Heat the garlic-infused oil in a large skillet over medium heat.
2. Add the shrimp and cook for 2-3 minutes, until they start to turn pink.
3. Pour in the white wine and lemon juice, and cook for another 2-3 minutes, until the shrimp are fully cooked.
4. Stir in the chopped parsley, and season with salt and pepper.

Practical Tip: Serve this shrimp scampi over a bed of steamed rice or gluten-free pasta for a complete meal.

3. Classic Steamed Mussels

Ingredients

- 2 pounds mussels, cleaned and debearded
- 1 tablespoon garlic-infused oil

- 1 cup dry white wine
- 1/2 cup chopped tomatoes (canned or fresh, seeds removed)
- 1/4 cup chopped fresh parsley
- Salt and pepper to taste

Instructions

1. Heat the garlic-infused oil in a large pot over medium heat.
2. Add the mussels, white wine, and tomatoes.
3. Cover and steam for 5-7 minutes, until the mussels open.
4. Discard any mussels that do not open.
5. Stir in the chopped parsley, and season with salt and pepper.

Practical Tip: Serve with gluten-free bread to soak up the delicious broth.

Low FODMAP Seafood Specials

Seared Scallops with Lemon Butter Sauce

Ingredients

- 1 pound large scallops, patted dry

- 2 tablespoons olive oil
- Salt and pepper to taste
- 2 tablespoons butter
- Juice of 1 lemon
- 2 tablespoons chopped fresh chives

Instructions

1. Heat olive oil in a large skillet over medium-high heat.
2. Season the scallops with salt and pepper.
3. Sear the scallops for 2-3 minutes per side, until they develop a golden-brown crust.
4. Remove scallops from the skillet and set aside.
5. Reduce heat to medium, add butter and lemon juice to the skillet, stirring until the butter melts and forms a sauce.
6. Return the scallops to the skillet, spooning the sauce over them.
7. Sprinkle with fresh chives before serving.

Practical Tip: Ensure your scallops are dry before searing to get a nice crust. Pat them with a paper towel if necessary.

2. Baked Cod with Puttanesca Sauce and Cherry Tomatoes

Ingredients

- 2 anchovy fillets, drained and chopped (optional)
- ½ teaspoon dried oregano
- Pinch of red pepper flakes (adjust to preference for heat)
- ½ cup cherry tomatoes, halved
- Chopped fresh parsley, for garnish

Instructions

1. Preheat oven to 400°F (200°C).
2. Pat the cod fillets dry with paper towels. Season both sides generously with salt and pepper.
3. In a large skillet, heat olive oil over medium heat. Add the chopped anchovy fillets (if using) and cook for 30 seconds, until they dissolve and release their flavor.
4. Pour in the diced tomatoes with their juices. Stir in the chopped Kalamata olives, capers, oregano, and red pepper flakes. Bring to a

simmer and cook for 5 minutes, allowing the flavors to meld.

5. Transfer the puttanesca sauce to a shallow baking dish. Nestle the seasoned cod fillets into the sauce.

6. Arrange the halved cherry tomatoes around the cod in the baking dish.

7. Bake for 15-20 minutes, or until the cod is cooked through and flaky. The cherry tomatoes should be softened and blistered.

8. Serve the baked cod with puttanesca sauce spooned over the top. Garnish with chopped fresh parsley.

Tip: Want to add a nutty flavor? Top the dish with a sprinkle of toasted pine nuts before serving.

While this recipe is low-FODMAP, remember that individual tolerances can vary. Start with a smaller portion of capers, as some individuals with IBS may be more sensitive to them. You can also adjust the amount of red pepper flakes based on your spice preference. Listen to your body and adjust the recipe as needed to manage your IBS symptoms.

Chapter 7: Meat Masterpieces

In this section, you'll discover a variety of scrumptious recipes featuring beef, pork, lamb, and more. Each recipe has been meticulously crafted to be Low FODMAP, ensuring that they are bursting with flavor while being gentle on your digestive system. This allows you to savor hearty, fulfilling meals without exacerbating your IBS symptoms.

Beef Dishes

Classic Beef Stir-Fry

Ingredients

- 1 lb. beef sirloin, thinly sliced
- 2 tbsp olive oil
- 1 red bell pepper, sliced
- 1 green bell pepper, sliced
- 1 carrot, julienned
- 1 zucchini, sliced
- 2 tbsp soy sauce (gluten-free)

- 1 tbsp rice vinegar
- 1 tsp grated ginger
- 1 tbsp sesame seeds
- 2 green onions, green parts only, chopped

Instructions

1. Heat 1 tbsp of olive oil in a large skillet over medium-high heat.
2. Add the beef slices and cook until browned, about 4-5 minutes. Remove and set aside.
3. In the same skillet, add the remaining olive oil and sauté the bell peppers, carrot, and zucchini until tender-crisp, about 5 minutes.
4. Return the beef to the skillet. Add soy sauce, rice vinegar, and ginger. Stir well to combine.
5. Cook for another 2-3 minutes, until the sauce thickens slightly.
6. Sprinkle with sesame seeds and green onions before serving. Enjoy with a side of rice or quinoa.

Tip: Make sure to slice the beef thinly against the grain for tender pieces.

2. Braised Beef Short Ribs with Red Wine and Shallots

Ingredients

- 2 tablespoons olive oil
- 2 pounds bone-in beef short ribs, trimmed
- 1 medium onion, chopped
- 4 shallots, peeled and halved
- 2 carrots, peeled and chopped
- 1 celery stalk, chopped
- 2 cloves garlic, minced
- 1 (750 ml) bottle low-FODMAP red wine
- 1 cup low-FODMAP beef broth
- 2 tablespoons tomato paste (check for low-FODMAP brands)
- 1 tablespoon chopped fresh thyme
- Salt and pepper to taste
- Chopped fresh parsley, for garnish (optional)

Instructions

1. Preheat oven to 325°F (165°C).
2. Heat olive oil in a large Dutch oven or oven-safe pot over medium-high heat. Season the beef short ribs generously with salt and pepper. Sear them on all sides until browned.

3. Remove the browned short ribs from the pot and set aside.

4. Add the chopped onion, shallots, carrots, and celery to the pot. Sauté for 5-7 minutes, or until softened.

5. Stir in the minced garlic and cook for an additional minute, allowing the aroma to bloom.

6. Pour in the red wine, scraping up any browned bits from the bottom of the pot. Bring to a simmer and cook for 5 minutes, allowing the alcohol to slightly reduce.

7. Add the beef broth, tomato paste, thyme, and additional salt and pepper to taste. Stir to combine.

8. Return the browned short ribs to the pot, ensuring they are submerged in the liquid. Bring to a boil, then cover the pot tightly.

9. Transfer the pot to the preheated oven and braise for 2-2 ½ hours, or until the beef is tender and falling off the bone.

10. Once cooked, remove the short ribs from the pot and shred the meat with two forks. Discard the bones.

11. Strain the braising liquid into a saucepan and skim off any excess fat from the surface. You can optionally thicken the sauce by simmering it over medium heat until it reduces slightly.

12. Return the shredded beef to the sauce and warm through.

13. Serve the braised beef short ribs with the sauce spooned over mashed potatoes, polenta, or low-FODMAP rice. Garnish with chopped fresh parsley (optional).

Tip: Want to add some vegetables? Include chopped mushrooms or green beans along with the other vegetables in step 4.

Pork Favorites

Honey Garlic Pork Chops

Ingredients

- 4 boneless pork chops
- 2 tbsp olive oil
- 2 tbsp honey
- 2 tbsp soy sauce (gluten-free)

- 1 tbsp rice vinegar
- 1 tsp garlic-infused olive oil
- 1 tsp dried thyme
- Salt and pepper to taste

Instructions

1. Season the pork chops with salt and pepper on both sides.
2. Heat olive oil in a large skillet over medium-high heat.
3. Add the pork chops and cook until browned and cooked through, about 4-5 minutes per side. Remove from the skillet and set aside.
4. In the same skillet, combine honey, soy sauce, rice vinegar, garlic-infused olive oil, and thyme. Stir and cook until the sauce begins to thicken, about 2-3 minutes.
5. Return the pork chops to the skillet and coat them with the sauce. Cook for an additional 1-2 minutes.
6. Serve the pork chops drizzled with the honey garlic sauce.

Tip: For extra flavor, marinate the pork chops in the sauce for at least 30 minutes before cooking.

2. Honey Garlic Glazed Pork Tenderloin with Roasted Brussels Sprouts

Ingredients

- 1 pork tenderloin (about 1-1.5 pounds)
- 1 tablespoon olive oil
- Salt and pepper to taste
- For the Honey Garlic Glaze:
    - ¼ cup low-FODMAP honey
    - 2 tablespoons soy sauce (check for low-FODMAP brands)
    - 1 tablespoon Dijon mustard
    - 1 clove garlic, minced
    - 1 tablespoon rice vinegar (check for low-FODMAP brands)
- 1 pound Brussels sprouts, trimmed and halved

Instructions

1. Preheat oven to 400°F (200°C).
2. Pat the pork tenderloin dry with paper towels.

Season generously with salt and pepper.

3. Heat olive oil in a large oven-safe skillet over medium-high heat. Sear the pork tenderloin on all sides until browned.

4. In a small bowl, whisk together the ingredients for the honey garlic glaze: honey, soy sauce, Dijon mustard, minced garlic, and rice vinegar.

5. Pour the glaze over the seared pork tenderloin in the skillet.

6. Toss the halved Brussels sprouts with a drizzle of olive oil, salt, and pepper. Arrange them around the pork tenderloin in the skillet.

7. Transfer the skillet to the preheated oven and bake for 20-25 minutes, or until the pork is cooked through and the Brussels sprouts are tender-crisp. Baste the pork with the glaze occasionally while baking.

8. Once cooked, remove the skillet from the oven and let the pork rest for 5 minutes before slicing.

Lamb and Other Meats

Herb-Crusted Lamb Chops

Ingredients

- 8 lamb chops
- 2 tbsp olive oil
- 2 tbsp fresh rosemary, chopped
- 2 tbsp fresh thyme, chopped
- 1 tsp garlic-infused olive oil
- Salt and pepper to taste
- Lemon wedges for serving

Instructions

1. Preheat the oven to 400°F (200°C).
2. In a small bowl, mix together the olive oil, rosemary, thyme, garlic-infused olive oil, salt, and pepper.
3. Rub the mixture onto both sides of the lamb chops.
4. Heat a large ovenproof skillet over medium-high heat. Add the lamb chops and sear for 2-3 minutes on each side until browned.
5. Transfer the skillet to the preheated oven and roast for 6-8 minutes for medium-rare, or

longer if you prefer.

6. Remove from the oven and let rest for a few minutes before serving with lemon wedges.

Tip: Letting the lamb chops rest before serving helps to retain their juices and flavor.

2. Moroccan Spiced Lamb Meatballs with Mint Yogurt Sauce

Ingredients

- 1 pound ground lamb
- ½ cup chopped onion
- ¼ cup chopped fresh parsley
- 2 tablespoons grated breadcrumbs (check for low-FODMAP bread)
- 1 teaspoon ground cumin
- ½ teaspoon ground coriander
- Pinch of ground cinnamon
- Salt and pepper to taste

For the Mint Yogurt Sauce:

- 1 cup plain whole milk yogurt (lactose-free option available)
- ¼ cup chopped fresh mint

- 1 tablespoon lemon juice
- Salt and pepper to taste

Instructions:

1. In a large bowl, combine ground lamb, chopped onion, parsley, breadcrumbs, cumin, coriander, cinnamon, salt, and pepper. Mix well with your hands to combine.
2. Form the mixture into small meatballs, about 1-inch in diameter.
3. Heat a large skillet with a drizzle of olive oil over medium heat. Add the meatballs and cook for 5-7 minutes, turning them occasionally, until browned on all sides.
4. While the meatballs cook, prepare the mint yogurt sauce. In a small bowl, whisk together yogurt, chopped fresh mint, lemon juice, salt, and pepper.
5. Once browned, reduce the heat to low and add a splash of water or low-FODMAP broth to the pan with the meatballs. Cover the pan and simmer for 5-7 minutes, or until the meatballs are cooked through.
6. Serve the Moroccan spiced lamb meatballs

warm with the mint yogurt sauce for dipping. Alternatively, serve them over a bed of low-FODMAP couscous drizzled with the sauce.

Tip: This recipe is already low-FODMAP, but remember to adjust portion sizes according to your individual tolerance. Start with a smaller portion of the mint yogurt sauce, as some individuals with IBS may be more sensitive to dairy. You can also use a lactose-free yogurt option if needed.

Practical Tips for Cooking Meat

1. Choose the Right Cut: Select tender cuts like sirloin, tenderloin, or chops for quick cooking methods. Tougher cuts like chuck or shoulder are better for slow cooking.

2. Season Well: Simple seasonings like salt, pepper, and herbs enhance the natural flavors of the meat.

3. Cook to the Right Temperature: Use a meat thermometer to ensure your meat is cooked to the right temperature. For beef, medium-rare is 135°F, and for pork, 145°F.

4. Rest the Meat: Let cooked meat rest for a few

minutes before slicing to keep it juicy.

Enjoy these meat masterpieces and make them a staple in your Low FODMAP diet!

Chapter 8: Vegetarian and Vegan Creations

Eating a vegetarian or vegan diet while following Low FODMAP guidelines might seem challenging, but it doesn't have to be. This chapter will show you how to create delicious plant-based meals that are both nutritious and gentle on your digestive system.

Plant-Based Meals

Creamy Coconut Curry with Vegetables and Chickpeas

Ingredients

- 1 tablespoon olive oil
- 1 medium onion, chopped
- 2 cloves garlic, minced

- 1 inch ginger, grated
- 1 tablespoon yellow curry powder
- 1 teaspoon ground cumin
- Pinch of red pepper flakes (adjust to preference for heat)
- 1 (14.5 oz) can diced tomatoes, undrained
- 1 (13.5 oz) can unsweetened coconut milk
- 1 cup low-FODMAP vegetable broth
- 1 cup chopped broccoli florets
- 1 cup sliced red bell pepper
- 1 (15 oz) can chickpeas, drained and rinsed
- Salt and pepper to taste
- Chopped fresh cilantro, for garnish (optional)
- Cooked brown rice or quinoa, for serving

Instructions

1. Heat olive oil in a large pot or Dutch oven over medium heat. Add the chopped onion and sauté for 5-7 minutes, or until softened.
2. Stir in the minced garlic and grated ginger. Cook for an additional minute, allowing the aromas to bloom.
3. Add the yellow curry powder, cumin, and red pepper flakes (start with a smaller amount and

adjust to your spice preference). Cook for 30 seconds, stirring constantly, to toast the spices.

4. Pour in the diced tomatoes with their juices. Scrape up any browned bits from the bottom of the pot.

5. Add the coconut milk, vegetable broth, broccoli florets, and sliced red bell pepper. Bring to a simmer and cook for 10-12 minutes, or until the vegetables are tender-crisp.

6. Stir in the drained and rinsed chickpeas. Season with salt and pepper to taste.

7. Let the curry simmer for an additional 5 minutes to allow the flavors to meld.

8. Serve the creamy coconut curry over cooked brown rice or quinoa. Garnish with chopped fresh cilantro (optional).

Tip: Want to add a protein boost? Marinate and sauté cubed tempeh or tofu for 15 minutes before adding it to the curry in step 6.

2. Lentil Shepherd's Pie with Creamy Cauliflower Mash

Ingredients

- 1 tablespoon olive oil

- 1 medium onion, chopped

- 2 carrots, peeled and diced

- 2 celery stalks, diced

- 2 cloves garlic, minced

- 1 teaspoon dried thyme

- 1 teaspoon dried rosemary

- 1 cup brown lentils, rinsed

- 4 cups low-FODMAP vegetable broth

- 1 (14.5 oz) can diced tomatoes, undrained

- 1 cup frozen peas

- Salt and pepper to taste

For the Creamy Cauliflower Mash:

- 1 head cauliflower, cut into florets

- ½ cup unsweetened almond milk

- 1 tablespoon olive oil

- Salt and pepper to taste

Instructions

1. Heat olive oil in a large pot or Dutch oven over medium heat. Add the chopped onion, carrots, and celery. Sauté for 5-7 minutes, or until softened.

2. Stir in the minced garlic, dried thyme, and

dried rosemary. Cook for an additional minute, allowing the aromas to bloom.

3. Add the rinsed brown lentils, vegetable broth, and diced tomatoes. Bring to a simmer and cook for 20-25 minutes, or until the lentils are tender.

4. While the lentils cook, prepare the creamy cauliflower mash. In a separate pot, steam the cauliflower florets until tender.

5. In a blender or food processor, combine the steamed cauliflower florets with almond milk, olive oil, salt, and pepper. Blend until smooth and creamy.

6. Once the lentils are cooked, stir in the frozen peas. Season with salt and pepper to taste.

7. Preheat oven to broil. Transfer the lentil mixture to a baking dish. Top with the creamy cauliflower mash, spreading it evenly.

8. Broil for 2-3 minutes, or until the top is golden brown and slightly bubbly.

9. Serve the lentil shepherd's pie warm with a sprinkle of fresh herbs (optional).

Tip: Want to add a protein boost? Top the shepherd's pie with a dollop of low-FODMAP yogurt or a sprinkle of chopped nuts.

3. Thai Coconut Curry Noodle Soup with Vegetables and Edamame

Ingredient

- 1 tablespoon olive oil
- 1 medium onion, chopped
- 2 cloves garlic, minced
- 1 inch ginger, grated
- 1 tablespoon yellow curry powder
- 1 teaspoon ground coriander
- Pinch of red pepper flakes (adjust to preference for heat)
- 1 (14.5 oz) can diced tomatoes, undrained
- 1 (13.5 oz) can unsweetened coconut milk
- 4 cups low-FODMAP vegetable broth

- 1 cup chopped broccoli florets
- 1 cup sliced red bell pepper
- 1 cup chopped green beans
- 8 oz rice noodles (check for low-FODMAP brands)
- 1 cup frozen shelled edamame, thawed
- Salt and pepper to taste
- Chopped fresh cilantro, for garnish (optional)
- Lime wedges, for serving

Instructions

1. Heat olive oil in a large pot or Dutch oven over medium heat. Add the chopped onion and sauté for 5-7 minutes, or until softened.
2. Stir in the minced garlic and grated ginger. Cook for an additional minute, allowing the aromas to bloom.
3. Add the yellow curry powder, coriander, and red pepper flakes. Cook for 30 seconds, stirring constantly, to toast the spices.
4. Pour in the diced tomatoes with their juices. Scrape up any browned bits from the bottom of the pot.
5. Add the coconut milk, vegetable broth,

broccoli florets, sliced red bell pepper, and green beans. Bring to a simmer and cook for 10-12 minutes, or until the vegetables are tender-crisp.

6. While the vegetables cook, cook the rice noodles according to package directions. Drain and rinse under cold water.

7. Add the thawed edamame to the simmering curry soup. Season with salt and pepper to taste.

8. To serve, divide the cooked rice noodles between bowls. Ladle the hot curry soup over the noodles. Garnish with chopped fresh cilantro (optional) and a squeeze of lime.

Tip: Want to add a protein boost? Top the soup with a sprinkle of toasted pumpkin seeds or chopped peanuts.

❖ Creative Tofu and Tempeh Dishes

Spicy Korean BBQ Tofu Bowls with Kimchi Slaw

Ingredients

- **For the Marinated Tofu:**
    - 1 block (14 oz) firm tofu, drained and pressed
    - ¼ cup low-FODMAP tamari sauce (or coconut aminos)
    - 1 tablespoon sesame oil
    - 1 tablespoon rice vinegar (check for low-FODMAP brands)
    - 1 tablespoon brown sugar
    - 1 clove garlic, minced
    - 1 teaspoon grated ginger
    - ½ teaspoon Korean chili flakes (adjust to preference for heat)
- **For the Kimchi Slaw:**
    - 1 cup chopped Napa cabbage
    - ½ cup shredded carrots
    - ¼ cup chopped scallions (green parts only)
    - 2 tablespoons low-FODMAP kimchi, chopped (adjust to preference for spice)
    - 1 tablespoon rice vinegar (check for low-FODMAP brands)
    - 1 teaspoon sesame oil
    - Salt and pepper to taste

- **For the Bowls:**
    - Cooked brown rice or quinoa
    - Chopped avocado
    - Toasted sesame seeds, for garnish

Instructions

1. **Marinate the Tofu:** Slice the drained and pressed tofu into bite-sized cubes.
2. In a shallow dish, whisk together tamari sauce, sesame oil, rice vinegar, brown sugar, minced garlic, grated ginger, and Korean chili flakes. Add the tofu cubes to the marinade and toss to coat them evenly. Let the tofu marinate for at least 30 minutes, or up to overnight for deeper flavor.
3. **Prepare the Kimchi Slaw:** In a bowl, combine chopped Napa cabbage, shredded carrots, scallions, chopped kimchi, rice vinegar, sesame oil, salt, and pepper. Toss to combine and let sit for at least 10 minutes to allow the flavors to meld.
4. **Cook the Tofu:** Heat a large skillet with a drizzle of oil over medium heat. Add the marinated tofu cubes and cook for 5-7 minutes

per side, or until golden brown and crispy.

5. **Assemble the Bowls:** Divide cooked brown rice or quinoa between bowls. Top with the cooked and crispy tofu cubes, kimchi slaw, chopped avocado, and a sprinkle of toasted sesame seeds.

Tip: Want to add a cooling element? Drizzle the bowls with a low-FODMAP sriracha mayo for a touch of creaminess and extra heat.

2. Spicy Korean BBQ Tempeh Lettuce Wraps with Miso Glaze

This is a flavorful and fun dish, it is a playful twist on another Korean BBQ, perfect for a light and healthy meal.

Ingredients:

- **For the Marinated Tempeh:**
  - 1 block (8 oz) tempeh, sliced into thin strips
  - ¼ cup low-FODMAP tamari sauce (or coconut aminos)
  - 1 tablespoon sesame oil
  - 1 tablespoon rice vinegar (check for low-

FODMAP brands)

- ○ 1 tablespoon brown sugar
- ○ 1 clove garlic, minced
- ○ 1 teaspoon grated ginger
- ○ ½ teaspoon Korean chili flakes (adjust to preference for heat)
- **For the Miso Glaze:**
  - ○ 2 tablespoons white miso paste
  - ○ 1 tablespoon rice vinegar (check for low-FODMAP brands)
  - ○ 1 tablespoon maple syrup
  - ○ 1 tablespoon water
- **For the Wraps:**
  - ○ 1 head romaine lettuce leaves, washed and dried
  - ○ Shredded carrots
  - ○ Chopped cucumber
  - ○ Pickled red onion (optional)
  - ○ Chopped fresh cilantro
  - ○ Toasted sesame seeds, for garnish

Instructions

1. **Marinate the Tempeh:** In a shallow dish, whisk together tamari sauce, sesame oil, rice

vinegar, brown sugar, minced garlic, grated ginger, and Korean chili flakes. Add the tempeh strips to the marinade and toss to coat them evenly. Let the tempeh marinate for at least 30 minutes, or up to overnight for deeper flavor.

2. **Prepare the Miso Glaze:** In a small bowl, whisk together white miso paste, rice vinegar, maple syrup, and water until smooth. Set aside.

3. **Cook the Tempeh:** Heat a large skillet with a drizzle of oil over medium heat. Add the marinated tempeh strips and cook for 5-7 minutes per side, or until golden brown and crispy.

4. **Assemble the Wraps:** Place a romaine lettuce leaf on a plate. Add a few strips of cooked tempeh, shredded carrots, chopped cucumber, pickled red onion (optional) , chopped fresh cilantro, and a drizzle of the miso glaze. Repeat with remaining ingredients to assemble more wraps.

5. Garnish with toasted sesame seeds.

Tip: Want to add a cooling element? Serve the wraps

with a side of low-FODMAP kimchi for a touch of spice and crunch.

❖ **Nutritious Vegetable Plates:**

Roasted Rainbow Vegetables with Lemon Herb Vinaigrette

Ingredients

- 1 head broccoli, cut into florets
- 1 head cauliflower, cut into florets
- 1 red bell pepper, sliced
- 1 yellow bell pepper, sliced
- 1 red onion, sliced
- 1 zucchini, sliced
- 2 tablespoons olive oil
- Salt and pepper to taste

For the Lemon Herb Vinaigrette:

- ¼ cup olive oil
- 2 tablespoons lemon juice
- 1 tablespoon balsamic vinegar (check for low-

FODMAP brands)

- 1 teaspoon dried oregano
- ½ teaspoon dried thyme
- Salt and pepper to taste

Instructions

1. Preheat oven to 400°F (200°C).
2. In a large bowl, toss the broccoli florets, cauliflower florets, sliced bell peppers, red onion, and zucchini with olive oil, salt, and pepper.
3. Spread the vegetables evenly on a large baking sheet.
4. Roast for 20-25 minutes, or until the vegetables are tender-crisp and slightly browned.
5. While the vegetables roast, prepare the lemon herb vinaigrette. In a small bowl, whisk together olive oil, lemon juice, balsamic vinegar, dried oregano, dried thyme, salt, and pepper.
6. Once the vegetables are roasted, remove them from the oven and let them cool slightly.
7. Transfer the roasted vegetables to a serving

platter and drizzle with the lemon herb vinaigrette. Toss to coat evenly.

Tip: Want to add a protein boost? Top the roasted vegetables with crumbled feta cheese or a sprinkle of roasted chickpeas.

2. Rainbow Veggie Skewers with Lemon Herb Marinade and Yogurt Dill Dip

Ingredients

- **For the Vegetable Skewers:**
    - 1 red bell pepper, cut into squares
    - 1 yellow bell pepper, cut into squares
    - 1 zucchini, cut into thick slices
    - 1 red onion, cut into wedges
    - 1 eggplant, cut into thick slices (optional)
    - 1 cup cherry tomatoes
    - 1 tablespoon olive oil
    - Salt and pepper to taste

- **For the Lemon Herb Marinade:**
    - ¼ cup olive oil

-     2 tablespoons lemon juice
-     1 tablespoon dried oregano
-     1 teaspoon dried thyme
-     1 clove garlic, minced
-     Pinch of red pepper flakes (adjust to preference for heat)
-     Salt and pepper to taste

- **For the Yogurt Dill Dip:**
  -     1 cup plain whole milk yogurt (lactose-free option available)
  -     ¼ cup chopped fresh dill
  -     1 tablespoon lemon juice
  -     Salt and pepper to taste

Instructions

1. **Prepare the Vegetables:** Wash and cut all vegetables according to the ingredient list. Ensure all pieces are similar in size for even cooking.

2. **Marinate the Vegetables:** In a shallow dish, whisk together olive oil, lemon juice, oregano, thyme, minced garlic, red pepper flakes (optional), salt, and pepper. Add the cut vegetables to the marinade and toss to coat

them evenly. Let the vegetables marinate for at least 30 minutes, or up to overnight for deeper flavor.

3. **Prepare the Yogurt Dill Dip:** In a small bowl, whisk together yogurt, chopped fresh dill, lemon juice, salt, and pepper. Cover and refrigerate until ready to serve.

4. **Assemble the Skewers:** Thread the marinated vegetables onto skewers, alternating colors for a visually appealing presentation. You can use wooden or metal skewers, pre-soaked if using wooden ones to prevent burning.

5. **Cooking Options:** You can grill the skewers over medium heat for 10-12 minutes per side, or until tender-crisp and slightly charred. Alternatively, preheat your oven to 400°F (200°C) and roast the skewers on a baking sheet for 20-25 minutes, flipping them halfway through cooking.

6. **Serve:** Serve the grilled or roasted vegetable skewers warm or at room temperature with the yogurt dill dip for dipping.

Tip: Want to add a protein element? Thread cooked shrimp or chicken cubes onto the skewers along with the vegetables.

While this recipe is already low-FODMAP, remember to listen to your body. Onions can be a trigger for some individuals with IBS. Start with a smaller amount of red onion or omit it entirely and substitute with another low-FODMAP vegetable like green beans or asparagus.

Chapter 9: Side Dishes and Accompaniments

When it comes to a well-rounded meal, side dishes and accompaniments play a crucial role. They complement the main dish and add variety, texture, and flavor to your plate. In this chapter, we'll explore a range of simple yet delicious Low FODMAP side dishes and accompaniments that you can easily incorporate into your meals.

Perfect Pairings

Roasted Carrots with Thyme

Ingredients

- 1 pound of carrots, peeled and cut into sticks
- 2 tablespoons olive oil
- 1 teaspoon dried thyme
- Salt and pepper to taste

Instructions

1. Preheat your oven to 400°F (200°C).
2. In a large bowl, toss the carrot sticks with olive oil, thyme, salt, and pepper.
3. Spread the carrots evenly on a baking sheet.
4. Roast in the oven for 20-25 minutes or until the carrots are tender and slightly caramelized.
5. Serve warm as a perfect side to any main dish.

Tip: For an extra flavor boost, add a sprinkle of lemon zest before serving.

Vegetables and Grains

Quinoa Pilaf with Vegetables

Ingredients

- 1 cup quinoa, rinsed
- 2 cups low FODMAP vegetable broth
- 1 tablespoon olive oil
- 1 red bell pepper, diced
- 1 zucchini, diced
- 1 cup baby spinach
- Salt and pepper to taste

Instructions

1. In a medium saucepan, bring the vegetable broth to a boil.
2. Add the rinsed quinoa, reduce the heat to low, cover, and simmer for about 15 minutes or until the quinoa is cooked and the broth is absorbed.
3. In a large skillet, heat the olive oil over medium heat.
4. Add the bell pepper and zucchini, and sauté for 5-7 minutes until the vegetables are tender.

5. Stir in the cooked quinoa and baby spinach. Cook for another 2-3 minutes until the spinach is wilted.

6. Season with salt and pepper to taste.

7. Serve warm as a nutritious side dish.

Tip: Make a big batch and use leftovers for a quick lunch the next day.

Flavorful Additions

Infused Oils and Vinegars

Ingredients

- For Garlic-Infused Olive Oil:
    - 1 cup extra virgin olive oil
    - 4 cloves garlic, peeled and lightly smashed
- For Rosemary-Infused Olive Oil:
    - 1 cup extra virgin olive oil
    - 2 sprigs fresh rosemary
- For Lemon-Infused Vinegar (check for low-FODMAP vinegar brands):
    - 1 cup white vinegar (check for low-FODMAP brands)

o   1 lemon, sliced

Instructions

1. **Garlic-Infused Olive Oil:** In a saucepan, combine olive oil and smashed garlic cloves. Heat gently over low heat for 10-15 minutes, never letting the oil simmer or boil. Remove from heat and let cool completely. Strain the garlic cloves from the oil. Store in an airtight container in a cool, dark place for up to 2 weeks.

2. **Rosemary-Infused Olive Oil:** Follow the same process as garlic-infused oil, substituting rosemary sprigs for garlic cloves.

3. **Lemon-Infused Vinegar:** In a saucepan, combine vinegar and sliced lemon. Heat gently over low heat for 10-15 minutes, never letting the vinegar simmer or boil. Remove from heat and let cool completely. Strain the lemon slices from the vinegar. Store in an airtight container in a cool, dark place for up to 2 weeks.

Tips:

- Experiment with different herbs and spices to create a variety of infused oils and vinegars. For example, try thyme, oregano, or chili flakes for infused olive oil, or orange or berries for infused vinegar (check for low-FODMAP options).
- Use infused oils for drizzling over roasted vegetables, grilled meats, or salads. Infused vinegars can be used in salad dressings, marinades, or deglazing pans.

If you have allergies to garlic or other ingredients used in infused oils, simply omit them and explore other flavor profiles. For example, consider using toasted nuts or seeds infused into the oil for a nutty and savory flavor.

These side dishes and accompaniments are designed to be simple, nutritious, and packed with flavor. They can easily be paired with a variety of main dishes to create a satisfying and balanced meal. Enjoy experimenting with these recipes and discovering your own favorite combinations

Chapter 10: Breads and Baked Goods

Baking your own Low FODMAP bread and baked goods can be incredibly rewarding. Not only do you get to enjoy fresh, delicious treats, but you also have complete control over the ingredients. In this chapter, we'll cover some essential recipes to get you started.

Low FODMAP Bread Recipes

1. Basic Low FODMAP bread

Ingredients

- 2 1/4 cups gluten-free flour blend
- 1 tsp xanthan gum (omit if your flour blend contains it)
- 1 1/2 tsp salt
- 1 tbsp sugar
- 1 packet (2 1/4 tsp) active dry yeast
- 1 cup warm water (110°F)
- 2 tbsp olive oil
- 2 eggs

Instructions

1. Preheat your oven to 375°F (190°C). Grease a loaf pan with olive oil.

2. In a large bowl, combine the gluten-free flour, xanthan gum (if needed), and salt.

3. In a separate bowl, mix the warm water and sugar, then sprinkle the yeast on top. Let it sit for about 5 minutes until it becomes frothy.

4. Add the olive oil and eggs to the yeast mixture and stir well.

5. Combine the wet ingredients with the dry ingredients. Mix until you have a smooth batter.

6. Pour the batter into the prepared loaf pan and smooth the top.

7. Let the dough rise in a warm place for about 30 minutes.

8. Bake for 35-40 minutes until the bread is golden brown and sounds hollow when tapped.

9. Let it cool completely before slicing.

2. Seeded Sunflower Seed Bread

Ingredients

- 1 ½ cups almond flour
- ½ cup psyllium husk powder
- ½ cup ground sunflower seeds
- ¼ cup chia seeds
- 2 teaspoons baking powder
- 1 teaspoon baking soda
- ½ teaspoon salt
- 3 tablespoons melted coconut oil
- 1 ½ cups unsweetened almond milk
- 2 large eggs
- ¼ cup chopped sunflower seeds (for topping)

Instructions

1. Preheat oven to 350°F (175°C). Grease a loaf pan.
2. In a large bowl, whisk together almond flour, psyllium husk powder, ground sunflower seeds, chia seeds, baking powder, baking soda, and salt.
3. In a separate bowl, whisk together melted coconut oil, almond milk, and eggs.
4. Pour the wet ingredients into the dry ingredients and stir until just combined. Be careful not to overmix.

5. Fold in the chopped sunflower seeds for topping.

6. Pour the batter into the prepared loaf pan and sprinkle with additional chopped sunflower seeds (optional).

7. Bake for 50-60 minutes, or until a toothpick inserted into the center comes out clean.

8. Let the bread cool in the pan for 10 minutes before transferring it to a wire rack to cool completely.

Tip: Want to add a touch of sweetness? Add a tablespoon of maple syrup or honey (check for low-FODMAP brands) to the wet ingredients.

Tip: Psyllium husk powder can be a source of gas for some individuals with IBS. Start with a smaller amount (¼ cup) and gradually increase if tolerated. You can also substitute psyllium husk powder with ground flaxseed meal.

Muffins, Scones, and More

1. Blueberry Muffins

Ingredients

- 2 cups gluten-free flour blend
- 2 tsp baking powder
- 1/2 tsp baking soda
- 1/4 tsp salt
- 1/2 cup sugar
- 1/4 cup melted butter
- 1/2 cup lactose-free yogurt
- 2 eggs
- 1 cup fresh or frozen blueberries

Instructions

1. Preheat your oven to 350°F (175°C). Line a muffin tin with paper liners.
2. In a large bowl, whisk together the flour, baking powder, baking soda, salt, and sugar.
3. In another bowl, mix the melted butter, lactose-free yogurt, and eggs.
4. Add the wet ingredients to the dry ingredients and stir until just combined.
5. Gently fold in the blueberries.
6. Divide the batter evenly among the muffin cups.

7. Bake for 20-25 minutes until a toothpick inserted into the center comes out clean.

8. Allow the muffins to cool in the pan for 5 minutes before transferring to a wire rack to cool completely.

2. Savory Cheddar Scones

Ingredients

- 2 cups gluten-free flour blend
- 1 tbsp baking powder
- 1/2 tsp salt
- 1/4 tsp garlic powder
- 1/4 tsp dried thyme
- 1/2 cup cold butter, cubed
- 1 cup shredded cheddar cheese
- 1/2 cup lactose-free milk

Instructions

1. Preheat your oven to 400°F (200°C). Line a baking sheet with parchment paper.

2. In a large bowl, combine the flour, baking powder, salt, garlic powder, and thyme.

3. Cut in the cold butter until the mixture resembles coarse crumbs.

4. Stir in the shredded cheddar cheese.

5. Gradually add the lactose-free milk, stirring until a dough forms.

6. Turn the dough out onto a floured surface and knead gently.

7. Pat the dough into a circle about 1 inch thick. Cut into 8 wedges and place them on the prepared baking sheet.

8. Bake for 15-20 minutes until the scones are golden brown.

9. Cool on a wire rack.

3. Low-FODMAP Banana Oat Muffins with Pecan Streusel

Ingredients

- **For the Muffins:**
    - 1 ½ cups rolled oats
    - ½ cup almond flour
    - ½ cup ground psyllium husk powder
    - 1 teaspoon baking powder
    - ½ teaspoon baking soda
    - ¼ teaspoon salt

- ○ 1 ripe banana, mashed
  - ○ 2 tablespoons melted coconut oil
  - ○ 1 cup unsweetened almond milk
  - ○ 2 large eggs
- **For the Pecan Streusel:**
  - ○ ¼ cup chopped pecans
  - ○ 2 tablespoons almond flour
  - ○ 1 tablespoon melted coconut oil
  - ○ Pinch of ground cinnamon

Instructions

1. Preheat oven to 375°F (190°C). Line a muffin tin with paper liners.
2. In a large bowl, whisk together rolled oats, almond flour, psyllium husk powder, baking powder, baking soda, and salt.
3. In a separate bowl, whisk together mashed banana, melted coconut oil, almond milk, and eggs.
4. Pour the wet ingredients into the dry ingredients and stir until just combined. Be careful not to overmix.
5. **Prepare the Pecan Streusel:** In a small bowl, combine chopped pecans, almond flour,

melted coconut oil, and ground cinnamon.

6. Divide the muffin batter evenly among the prepared muffin cups. Sprinkle each muffin with the pecan streusel topping.

7. Bake for 20-25 minutes, or until a toothpick inserted into the center comes out clean.

8. Let the muffins cool in the tin for a few minutes before transferring them to a wire rack to cool completely.

Tip: Want to add a touch of fruit? Fold in a handful of chopped blueberries or cranberries to the batter.

Delicious Desserts

Chocolate Chip Cookies

Ingredients

- 1 1/4 cups gluten-free flour blend
- 1/2 tsp baking soda
- 1/2 tsp salt
- 1/2 cup unsalted butter, softened

- 1/2 cup brown sugar
- 1/4 cup granulated sugar
- 1 egg
- 1 tsp vanilla extract
- 1 cup low FODMAP chocolate chips

Instructions

1. Preheat your oven to 350°F (175°C). Line a baking sheet with parchment paper.
2. In a medium bowl, whisk together the flour, baking soda, and salt.
3. In a large bowl, beat the softened butter, brown sugar, and granulated sugar until creamy.
4. Add the egg and vanilla extract and mix well.
5. Gradually add the dry ingredients to the wet ingredients and mix until combined.
6. Fold in the low FODMAP chocolate chips.
7. Drop rounded tablespoons of dough onto the prepared baking sheet.
8. Bake for 10-12 minutes until the edges are golden brown.
9. Allow the cookies to cool on the baking sheet for 5 minutes before transferring to a wire rack

to cool completely.

Tips:

- Always check the ingredients for FODMAP content. Gluten-free flour blends can vary, so ensure yours is low FODMAP.
- Measure your ingredients accurately, especially when baking gluten-free, as it can be less forgiving than regular baking.
- Allow baked goods to cool completely before slicing or serving to ensure the best texture.

2. Low-FODMAP Chocolate Chip Cookie Bars

Ingredients

- ¼ cup ground flaxseed meal
- ½ teaspoon baking soda
- ¼ teaspoon salt
- 6 tablespoons melted coconut oil
- ⅓ cup maple syrup (check for low-FODMAP brands)
- 2 large eggs
- 1 teaspoon vanilla extract
- ½ cup chopped dark chocolate chips (check for

low-FODMAP brands)

Instructions

1. Preheat oven to 350°F (175°C). Line an 8x8 inch baking pan with parchment paper.
2. In a large bowl, whisk together almond flour, rolled oats, cocoa powder, ground flaxseed meal, baking soda, and salt.
3. In a separate bowl, whisk together melted coconut oil, maple syrup, eggs, and vanilla extract.
4. Pour the wet ingredients into the dry ingredients and stir until just combined. Be careful not to overmix.
5. Fold in the chopped dark chocolate chips.
6. Pour the batter into the prepared baking pan and spread evenly.
7. Bake for 20-25 minutes, or until the edges are set and the center is slightly gooey.
8. Let the cookie bars cool completely in the pan before cutting into squares.

Tip: Want to add a sprinkle of salt? A pinch of flaky

sea salt on top of the warm bars adds a delicious sweet and salty contrast.

Enjoy these recipes and make your kitchen a place where delicious, IBS-friendly baked goods are always on the menu!

Chapter 11: Sauces and Condiments

Homemade Sauces

Low FODMAP Tomato Sauce

Ingredients

- 2 tbsp garlic-infused olive oil (use the oil only, discard the garlic)
- 1 can (14.5 oz) diced tomatoes (no added onion or garlic)
- 1 tbsp tomato paste
- 1 tsp dried basil
- 1 tsp dried oregano
- 1 tsp sugar
- Salt and pepper to taste

Instructions

1. Heat the garlic-infused olive oil in a saucepan over medium heat.
2. Add the diced tomatoes and tomato paste, stirring to combine.
3. Stir in the dried basil, oregano, and sugar.
4. Bring to a simmer and let cook for 20-30 minutes, stirring occasionally.
5. Season with salt and pepper to taste.
6. Use immediately or store in the refrigerator for up to a week.

Tip: If you prefer a smoother sauce, blend it using an immersion blender or a regular blender after it has cooled slightly.

2. Creamy Roasted Garlic and Herb Tahini Sauce

Ingredients

- 1 head garlic
- 2 tablespoons olive oil
- ½ cup tahini
- ¼ cup lemon juice
- ¼ cup water

- 1 tablespoon chopped fresh parsley
- 1 tablespoon chopped fresh dill
- ½ teaspoon dried oregano
- Salt and pepper to taste

Instructions

1. Preheat oven to 400°F (200°C).
2. **Roast the Garlic:** Cut the top off the head of garlic to expose the cloves. Drizzle with olive oil and wrap tightly in aluminum foil. Roast in the preheated oven for 40-45 minutes, or until the garlic cloves are soft and golden brown. Let cool slightly.
3. **Squeeze the Roasted Garlic:** Once cool enough to handle, squeeze the roasted garlic cloves out of their skins. You should have about 4-5 tablespoons of roasted garlic pulp.
4. **Blend the Sauce:** In a blender or food processor, combine roasted garlic pulp, tahini, lemon juice, water, chopped parsley, chopped dill, dried oregano, salt, and pepper. Blend until smooth and creamy. Add a little more water if needed to achieve desired consistency.
5. Taste and adjust seasonings as needed.

Tip: Want to add a kick of spice? Add a pinch of red pepper flakes to the blender with the other ingredients.

3. Low FODMAP Pesto

Ingredients

- 2 cups fresh basil leaves
- 1/4 cup pine nuts
- 1/2 cup grated Parmesan cheese
- 1/2 cup garlic-infused olive oil
- 1 tsp lemon juice
- Salt and pepper to taste

Instructions

1. In a food processor, combine the basil leaves, pine nuts, and Parmesan cheese.
2. Pulse until the mixture is finely chopped.
3. With the food processor running, slowly pour in the garlic-infused olive oil until the mixture is smooth.
4. Add lemon juice and season with salt and pepper to taste.

5. Store in an airtight container in the refrigerator for up to a week.

Tip: Pesto can be frozen in ice cube trays for easy, portioned use in future meals.

❖ Dressings and Dips

Low FODMAP Ranch Dressing

Ingredients

- 1 cup lactose-free plain yogurt
- 1/4 cup mayonnaise
- 2 tbsp garlic-infused olive oil
- 1 tbsp chopped fresh chives
- 1 tbsp chopped fresh dill
- 1 tbsp chopped fresh parsley
- 1 tsp lemon juice
- Salt and pepper to taste

Instructions

1. In a bowl, whisk together the lactose-free yogurt, mayonnaise, and garlic-infused olive oil until smooth.

2. Stir in the fresh chives, dill, and parsley.

3. Add the lemon juice and season with salt and pepper to taste.

4. Store in an airtight container in the refrigerator for up to a week.

Tip: This dressing can also double as a dip for vegetables or low FODMAP crackers.

2. Spicy Mango Habanero Vinaigrette

Ingredients

- 1 ripe mango, peeled and chopped
- 1/2 habanero pepper, seeded and chopped (adjust to preference for heat)
- 2 tablespoons olive oil
- 2 tablespoons lime juice
- 1 tablespoon rice vinegar (check for low-FODMAP brands)
- 1 tablespoon chopped fresh cilantro
- Salt and pepper to taste

Instructions

1. In a blender or food processor, combine chopped mango, habanero pepper (remove

seeds for less heat), olive oil, lime juice, rice vinegar, and chopped fresh cilantro.

2. Blend until smooth. Season with salt and pepper to taste.

3. Strain the vinaigrette through a fine-mesh sieve to remove any large pieces of mango or habanero pepper.

Tip: Want to add a creamy element? Whisk in a tablespoon of low-fat yogurt or sour cream before serving.

3. Low FODMAP Hummus

Ingredients

- 1 can (15 oz) chickpeas, drained and rinsed
- 2 tbsp garlic-infused olive oil
- 1/4 cup tahini
- 2 tbsp lemon juice
- 1/2 tsp ground cumin
- Salt and pepper to taste
- Water, as needed

Instructions

1. In a food processor, combine the chickpeas,

garlic-infused olive oil, tahini, lemon juice, and ground cumin.

2. Blend until smooth, adding water a tablespoon at a time to reach the desired consistency.

3. Season with salt and pepper to taste.

4. Store in an airtight container in the refrigerator for up to a week.

Tip: For extra flavor, sprinkle some smoked paprika or chopped fresh herbs on top before serving.

Flavor Enhancers

Low FODMAP Herb Butter

Ingredients

- 1/2 cup unsalted butter, softened
- 2 tbsp chopped fresh parsley
- 1 tbsp chopped fresh chives
- 1 tsp lemon zest
- Salt to taste

Instructions

1. In a bowl, combine the softened butter, fresh parsley, chives, and lemon zest.

2. Mix until well combined.

3. Add salt to taste.

4. Transfer to a piece of plastic wrap, shape into a log, and wrap tightly.

5. Refrigerate until firm, about 1 hour.

6. Slice and use as needed.

Tip: Herb butter can be frozen for up to three months. Just slice off what you need and keep the rest frozen.

2. Low FODMAP Teriyaki Sauce

Ingredients

- 1/4 cup soy sauce (ensure it's gluten-free if necessary)
- 1/4 cup water
- 2 tbsp brown sugar
- 1 tbsp rice vinegar
- 1 tbsp garlic-infused olive oil
- 1 tsp grated fresh ginger
- 1 tbsp cornstarch mixed with 1 tbsp water

Instructions

1. In a small saucepan, combine the soy sauce, water, brown sugar, rice vinegar, garlic-infused olive oil, and grated ginger.

2. Bring to a boil over medium heat, stirring occasionally.

3. Reduce the heat and let simmer for 5 minutes.

4. Stir in the cornstarch mixture and cook until the sauce thickens, about 2-3 minutes.

5. Remove from heat and let cool.

6. Store in an airtight container in the refrigerator for up to two weeks.

Tip: This sauce is perfect for marinating meats or drizzling over stir-fried vegetables and rice.

By incorporating these sauces and condiments into your meals, you can add a burst of flavor while keeping your diet Low FODMAP-friendly. Experiment with these recipes and enjoy the variety they bring to your dishes!

Bonus: 4-week Meal Plan

Managing IBS and sticking to a Low FODMAP diet can be challenging, but having a structured meal plan can make it much easier. This 30-day meal plan is designed to help you get started, explore a variety of recipes, refine your diet based on personal tolerance, and maintain a balanced diet long-term. Each week focuses on different aspects of the diet, ensuring you have a comprehensive and enjoyable experience.

Week 1: Getting Started

- Breakfast: Start your day with a Low FODMAP smoothie made with lactose-free yogurt, spinach, banana (limited to 1/3 of a ripe banana), and a handful of strawberries. Another great option is scrambled eggs with spinach and a slice of Low FODMAP toast.
- Lunch: Keep it simple with a chicken and quinoa salad. Use grilled chicken breast, cooked quinoa, mixed greens, cucumber, and a Low FODMAP dressing. For another option, try a tuna salad with lettuce, tomatoes, and a small amount of mayonnaise.
- Dinner: opt for grilled salmon with a side of steamed carrots and zucchini. Another idea is a simple stir-fry with chicken, bell peppers, and Bok choy served over rice.
- Snacks: Snack on Low FODMAP fruits like kiwi or oranges. You can also enjoy rice cakes

with peanut butter or a handful of almonds.

Week 2: Exploring More Recipes

Incorporating Variety and New Recipes

- Breakfast: Try overnight oats made with lactose-free milk, chia seeds, and blueberries. You can also enjoy a vegetable omelet with tomatoes, bell peppers, and spinach.
- Lunch: Experiment with a lentil soup made with Low FODMAP vegetables like carrots, celery, and tomatoes. Another option is a turkey and avocado wrap using a gluten-free tortilla.
- Dinner: Explore international flavors with dishes like Low FODMAP chicken tikka masala served with basmati rice. Alternatively, make a beef stir-fry with ginger, garlic, and mixed vegetables.
- Snacks: Enjoy carrot sticks with hummus or a small bowl of lactose-free yogurt with a drizzle of maple syrup.

Week 3: Refining Your Diet

Adjusting Meals Based on Personal Tolerance

By week three, you should start to identify which foods you tolerate well and which you don't. Use this week to refine your diet and make adjustments based on your tolerance.

- Breakfast: If you've found certain fruits more tolerable, incorporate them into your morning smoothies or cereal. For example, try a smoothie with pineapple and spinach or oatmeal with a sliced banana.
- Lunch: Adjust your salads and sandwiches based on what works best for you. If you tolerate tomatoes well, add them to your salads or sandwiches. If not, substitute with cucumber or bell peppers.
- Dinner: Focus on meals that have worked well for you so far. If chicken dishes have been gentle on your stomach, try a new recipe like chicken fajitas with bell peppers and a gluten-free tortilla.
- Snacks: Continue with snacks that you enjoy

and tolerate well. Make your Low FODMAP trail mix with nuts, seeds, and dried cranberries.

Week 4: Maintaining a Balanced Diet

Ensuring Long-Term Adherence and Satisfaction

- Breakfast: Make a batch of Low FODMAP muffins to have on hand for quick breakfasts. Pair them with a piece of fruit or a smoothie.

- Lunch: Prepare larger batches of your favorite Low FODMAP soups or salads to have ready for the week. This can save time and ensure you always have a healthy option available.

- Dinner: Continue to explore new recipes and adapt old favorites. Try a Low FODMAP pasta dish with a homemade tomato sauce and ground turkey or a baked potato with lactose-free sour cream and chives.

- Snacks: Keep various snacks on hand, such as fresh fruit, rice cakes, and nut butter. This will help you stay satisfied and avoid the temptation of high-FODMAP foods.

Conclusion

As you continue your Low FODMAP journey, stay patient and trust the process, surround yourself with supportive friends, family, community, and healthcare professionals who can provide guidance and encouragement along the way. I recommend you revisit this cookbook often, try new recipes, and share your experiences with others who may benefit from the Low FODMAP diet. Your journey can inspire and help those seeking relief from IBS.

Appendices

Appendix A: Low FODMAP Food Lists

High FODMAP Foods to Avoid

1. Fruits: Apples, cherries, mangoes, watermelon.

2. Vegetables: Asparagus, cauliflower, mushrooms, onions, garlic.

3. Dairy: Milk, soft cheeses, yogurt.

4. Grains: Wheat-based products, rye, barley.

5. Legumes: Baked beans, chickpeas, lentils.

6. Sweeteners: High fructose corn syrup, honey, agave nectar.

7. Beverages: Fruit juices, beer, sweetened drinks.

Low FODMAP Foods to Enjoy

1. Fruits: Bananas, blueberries, strawberries, oranges.

2. Vegetables: Carrots, cucumbers, eggplant, spinach, zucchini.

3. Dairy: Lactose-free milk, hard cheeses, butter.

4. Grains: Rice, oats, quinoa, gluten-free bread.

5. Proteins: Chicken, beef, fish, eggs, tofu (firm).

6. Nuts and Seeds: Almonds (small quantities), chia seeds, pumpkin seeds.

7. Beverages: Water, tea, coffee (in moderation).

Appendix B: Meal Planning Tips

1. Start Simple: Begin with basic recipes and gradually try more complex dishes.

2. Batch Cooking: Prepare larger quantities and freeze portions for future meals.

3. Diversify Your Diet: Rotate different foods to ensure balanced nutrition and avoid monotony.

4. Use Fresh Ingredients: Fresh produce often has better flavor and nutritional value.

5. Read Labels: Check food labels for hidden FODMAPs and ingredients that might trigger symptoms.

6. Stay Organized: Keep a well-organized pantry and refrigerator with Low FODMAP staples.

Appendix C: Frequently Asked Questions (FAQs)

What is the Low FODMAP Diet?

The Low FODMAP diet is a dietary approach designed to help manage symptoms of IBS by limiting foods high in specific types of carbohydrates that are difficult to digest.

How Long Should I Follow the Low FODMAP Diet?

Typically, the diet is followed strictly for 4-6 weeks, followed by a reintroduction phase to identify individual triggers.

Can I Eat Out While on the Low FODMAP Diet?

Yes, but it requires careful planning. Choose restaurants that offer customizable options, and don't hesitate to ask about ingredients and preparation methods.

Are There Any Risks Associated with the Low FODMAP Diet?

The diet can be restrictive, so it's important to ensure you're getting enough nutrients. Consult with a healthcare professional or dietitian for personalized guidance.

Appendix D: Resources for Further Reading

1. Books:

  - "The Complete Low-FODMAP Diet" by Sue Shepherd and Peter Gibson

  - "The Low-FODMAP Cookbook" by Dianne Fastenow Benjamin

  - "The IBS Elimination Diet" by Patsy Catsos

2. Websites:

  -    Monash   University   FODMAP: www.monashfodmap.com

  -    FODMAP   every   day: www.fodmapeveryday.com

3. Apps:

  - Monash University FODMAP Diet App

  - FODMAP Friendly App

Appendix F: Glossary of Terms

1.   FODMAPs: Fermentable Oligosaccharides, Disaccharides, Monosaccharides, and Polyols.

2. IBS: Irritable Bowel Syndrome, a digestive disorder causing symptoms like pain, bloating, and irregular bowel movements.

3. Monash University: The Australian university that developed the Low FODMAP diet.

4. Fructose: A simple sugar found in many fruits and honey.

5. Lactose: A sugar found in milk and dairy products.

6. Gluten: A protein found in wheat, barley, and rye.

7. Probiotics: Live bacteria and yeasts that are beneficial for digestive health.

8. Prebiotics: Types of fiber that feed the good bacteria in your gut.

9. Polyols: Sugar alcohols found in some fruits and artificial sweeteners.

Appendix G: Index

A

- Appetizers: Chapter 3

B

- Baked Goods: Chapter 10

- Birth : Chapter 1

- Beef Dishes: Chapter 7